The GP's Guide to Professional and Private Work Outside the NHS

Edited by

FRANK McKENNA

Head of Private Practice and Professional Fees
British Medical Association

and

DAVID PICKERSGILL

Chairman, Private Practice and Professional Fees Committee
British Medical Association

Foreword by

MAC ARMSTRONG

Secretary
British Medical Association

RADCLIFFE MEDICAL PRESS
OXFORD and NEW YORK

© 1995 Frank McKenna and David Pickersgill

Radcliffe Medical Press Ltd
18 Marcham Road, Abingdon, Oxon OX14 1AA, UK

Radcliffe Medical Press, Inc.
141 Fifth Avenue, New York, NY 10010, USA

Reprinted 1995

British Library Cataloguing in Publication Data

A catalogue record for this book is available from the British Library.

ISBN 1 85775 074 8

Library of Congress Cataloging-in-Publication Data is available.

Typeset by Marksbury Typesetting Ltd, Midsomer Norton, Avon.
Printed and bound by Redwood Books, Trowbridge, Wiltshire.

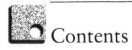 Contents

The GP's Guide to Professional and Private Work Outside the NHS

List of contributors

TIM ALBERT, *Medical Journalist, Castlebank House, Oak Road, Leatherhead, Surrey KT22 7PG*

ANGELA ANSTEY, *Solicitor, BMA Legal Department, BMA House, Tavistock Square, London WC1H 9JP*

STUART CARNE, *Vice President QPR Football Club, Past President RCGP, 5 St Mary Abbots Court, Warwick Gardens, London W14 8RA*

HUGH DE LA HAYE DAVIES, *President, Association of Police Surgeons, Creaton House, Creaton, Northampton, NN6 8ND*

BRIAN ELVY, *General Practitioner, Oak Street Medical Practice, Norwich NR3 3DL*

CHRIS EVANS, *Consultant Chest Physician and Chief Medical Advisor, Royal Life Company (Liverpool); The Cardiothoracic Centre, Liverpool, NHS Trust, Thomas Drive, Liverpool L14 3PE*

ERIC GODFREY, *General Practitioner and former part-time prison doctor, 2 Deplesdon Road, Cheadle, Stockport, Cheshire SK8 1DZ*

ROGER HARRINGTON, *General Practitioner and Secretary, Medical Officers for Schools Association, North End Surgery, High Street, Buckingham MK18 1NU*

EDDIE JOSSE, *General Practitioner, Brownlow Medical Centre, 140–142 Brownlow Road, London N11 2BD*

JOE KEARNS, *Consultant Occupational Physician, 9 Ascott Avenue, London W5 3XL*

SPENCER LEIGH, *Chief Underwriter, Royal Life Company, Liverpool*

ADRIAN MIDGLEY, *General Practitioner, The Homefield Surgery, Homefield Road, Exeter EX1 2QS*

GEOFFREY SAMSON, *Private General Practitioner, 80 Redcliffe Gardens, London SW10 9HE*

FRANK WELLS, *Director of Medicine, Science and Technology, Association of the British Pharmaceutical Industry, 12 Whitehall, London SW1A 2DY*

Editors

FRANK MCKENNA, *Head of Private Practice and Professional Fees, British
Medical Association, Tavistock Square, London WC1H 9JP*
DR DAVID PICKERSGILL, *Chairman, Private Practice and Professional Fees
Committee, British Medical Association, Tavistock Square, London
WC1H 9JP*

The Business Side of General Practice

Editorial board for the series

STUART CARNE, *former President, Royal College of General Practitioners*

JOHN CHISHOLM, *Joint Deputy Chairman and Negotiator, General Medical Services Committee, British Medical Association*

NORMAN ELLIS, *Under Secretary, British Medical Association*

EILEEN FARRANT, *former Chairman, Association of Medical Secretaries, Practice Administrators and Receptionists*

SANDRA GOWER, *Fellow Member of the Association of Managers in General Practice*

WILLIAM KENT, *Secretary, General Medical Services Committee, British Medical Association*

CLIVE PARR, *General Manager, Hereford and Worcester Family Health Services Authority*

DAVID TAYLOR, *Head of Health Care Quality, Audit Commission*

CHARLES ZUCKERMAN, *Secretary, Birmingham Local Medical Committee; Member, General Medical Services Committee, British Medical Association*

Foreword

GPs are being presented with ever increasing opportunities to undertake work outside their NHS contract. Some are well versed in how to develop the financial benefits these opportunities can bring to their practice. But others, not surprisingly, are unsure where to turn for information on how to develop these areas of work.

This book contains valuable advice and information on the practicalities of professional and private work outside the NHS. It draws on the knowledge and experience of both professional advisers and GPs themselves. I am confident that both newly appointed and experienced GPs alike will find this book informative, practical and essential reading if they wish to keep informed of professional opportunities outside the NHS.

Mac Armstrong
Secretary
British Medical Association
September 1995

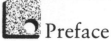 Preface

The opportunities for general practitioners to engage in both professional and private work have increased considerably in recent years. This book, for the first time, brings together some of the most common opportunities available to GPs who are considering ways of both maximizing their non-NHS earnings as well as stimulating and developing their clinical knowledge. Bringing together the wide-ranging areas covered by this book has been a challenging exercise and we are deeply indebted to the authors who have contributed to this book, both for their expertise in the relevant areas and for the commitment they have shown in meeting tight editing deadlines.

We are grateful to Mac Armstrong, BMA Secretary for writing the foreword, to Lyn Saywell, executive officer to the BMA's Private Practice and Professional Fees Committee, for comments on various chapters, to Angela Anstey, solicitor, BMA legal department, for comments on chapter 14 and to Norman Ellis, under secretary, BMA, for his support and guidance. Rosemary Topping and Helena Morris also deserve a vote of thanks for all their efforts in word processing various chapters. Finally, Gillian Nineham, Camilla Behrens and Kathryn Shellswell at Radcliffe Medical Press have been of enormous help and encouragement throughout the whole process of bringing this project together and we owe them our thanks.

Frank McKenna
David Pickersgill
September 1995

1   Everyday work for GPs outside the NHS contract

David Pickersgill

A working day can scarcely go by for the average GP without being asked to undertake some form of patient service that is outside the scope of the GP's contract with the NHS. Not only is this contract poorly understood by the public, but also it is often misunderstood by GPs themselves. This can lead to confusion about which services should be provided free of charge and, more importantly, when it is acceptable to charge a patient for a particular service. Happily, the NHS (General Medical Services) Regulations are quite explicit about which services must be provided free of charge (see paragraph 12 of the GMS Regulations).

Types of private service

The requests that GPs receive in their surgery to provide private services fall into two types; the provision of a certificate or written report, and a request to undertake an examination and then provide a written report, which may or may not also involve expressing an opinion. The information is often required in order for the patient to gain access to a State benefit, for the submission of claims in connection with various types of insurance or to confirm that the patient is medically fit to undertake some particular activity.

Much of the work has a high 'irritation' factor, patients often demanding the immediate completion of notes or certificates during time that the doctor has set aside for NHS consultations, and not infrequently for matters that are entirely unrelated to the patient's need for treatment. Doctors are, of course, free to refuse to undertake work of this type, but this almost inevitably leads to confrontation with patients, many of whom feel that doctors' NHS contracts require them to provide for the patient, whatever the patient demands. The patient (and some doctors) frequently fails to understand the legal implications of signing various certificates and statements, and prudent GPs should always pause and carefully consider what is being signed and whether they are truly in a position to make that particular statement about that patient. This is particularly important in connection with, for example, signing applications for shotgun licences, certificates of fitness to drive and certificates of fitness to undertake hazardous sporting activities. The doctor could easily find himself legally liable if he has certified an elderly patient fit to drive if that person is subsequently involved in an accident that is shown to be due to some aspect of the patient's health, such as failing eyesight or loss of mobility; making adequate control of the vehicle difficult.

Another matter for consideration is whether, by always acceding to patients' requests for private notes and certificates, doctors in general are making a rod for their own backs in terms of increasing work-load and patient expectation. Some employers make unreasonable demands of their employees always to obtain a private certificate from a doctor for minor self-limiting illnesses that have not required medical intervention. Some schools and teachers instruct parents to obtain a certificate from a doctor to cover children's absence from school or to confirm that they should be excused from gym or sporting activities. Our professional negotiators fought long and hard to remove the statutory requirements for short-term certification by doctors, and we, as GPs, should not allow ourselves to be forced back into this practice simply because a fee may be charged for work that we know in our hearts is unnecessary and wasteful of our time and skills.

Are doctors entitled to charge?

All registered doctors are obliged by statute to provide death certificates and stillbirth certificates without charge. Doctors in relevant posts are obliged by statute to provide certain services for which they are remunerated:

- infectious disease notification

- professional evidence in court when directed

- post mortems (when directed by the coroner).

The NHS terms of service for GPs impose certain contractual requirements on them. Paragraph 12 of the terms of service states 'That a doctor shall render to his patients all necessary and appropriate personal medical services of the type usually provided by general medical practitioners'. These services are further defined in that same paragraph:

12.2 The services which a doctor is required by sub-paragraph (1) to render shall include the following:

(a) giving advice, where appropriate, to a patient in connection with the patient's general health, and in particular about the significance of diet, exercise, the use of tobacco, the consumption of alcohol and the misuse of drugs or solvents;

(b) offering to patients consultations and, where appropriate, physical examinations for the purpose of identifying, or reducing the risk of, disease or injury;

(c) offering to patients, where appropriate, vaccination or immunisation against measles, mumps, rubella, pertussis, poliomyelitis, diphtheria and tetanus;

(d) arranging for the referral of patients, as appropriate, for the provision of any other services under the Act; and

(e) giving advice, as appropriate, to enable patients to avail themselves of services provided by a local social services authority.

In addition to the services that have to be provided to patients free of charge, the terms of service also contain, in Schedule 9, a list of prescribed medical certificates that must be provided free of charge (Table 1.1).

Table 1.1: Schedule 9 – list of prescribed medical certificates

Description of medical certificate	Short title of enactment under or for the purpose of which certificate required
1 To support a claim or obtain payment either personally or by proxy; to prove inability to work or incapacity for self-support for the purposes of an award by the Secretary of State; or to enable proxy to draw pensions etc	Naval and Marine Pay and Pensions Act 1865(a) Air Force (Constitution) Act 1917(b) Pensions (Navy, Army, Air Force and Mercantile Marine) Act 1939(c) Personal Injuries (Emergency Provisions) Act 1939(d) Pensions (Mercantile Marine) Act 1942(e) Polish Resettlement Act 1947(f) Home Guard Act 1951(g) Social Security Act 1975(h) Industrial Injuries and Diseases (Old Cases) Act 1975(i) Parts I and III of the Social Security and Housing Benefits Act 1982(j) Part II of, and Part V of, and Schedule 4 to, the Social Security Act 1986(k)
2 To establish pregnancy for the purpose of obtaining welfare foods	Section 13 of the Social Security Act 1988(1)
3 To establish fitness to receive inhalational analgesia in childbirth	Nurses, Midwives and Health Visitors Act 1979(m)

4	To secure registration of stillbirth	Births and Deaths Registration Act 1953(n)
5	To enable payment to be made to an institution or other person in case of mental disorder of persons entitled to payment from public funds	Section 142 of the Mental Health Act 1983(o)
6	To establish fitness for jury service	Juries Act 1974(p)
7	To establish unfitness to attend for medical examination	National Service Act 1948(q)
8	To support late application for reinstatement in civil employment or notification of non-availability to take up employment, owing to sickness	Reinstatement in Civil Employment Act 1944(r) Reinstatement in Civil Employment Act 1950(s) Reserve Forces Act 1980(t)
9	To enable a person to be registered as an absent voter on grounds of physical incapacity	Representation of the People Act 1983
10	To support application for certificates conferring exemption from charges in respect of drugs, medicines and appliances	National Health Service Act 1977
11	To support a claim by or on behalf of a severely mentally impaired person for exemption from liability to pay the community charge	Local Government Finance Act 1988

Also provided free of charge are certificates for patients claiming sickness and disability benefits, including Incapacity Benefit, Statutory Sick Pay, Disabled Living Allowance and Attendance Allowance, and replies to the Regional Medical Service on form RM2. Doctors may charge a fee for social security claims in relation to the Income Support scheme and the Social Fund. In relation to the former list of benefits, certificates must be issued free of charge for initial claims but not in connection with appeals and subsequent reviews, for which GPs can charge a fee for supplying letters or reports in support of these claims.

Private work in NHS hospitals

Doctors who work in hospitals (which also applies to GPs who hold clinical assistant or hospital practitioner posts) are subject to a separate set of terms of service, (the Hospital Medical and Dental Staff terms and conditions of service). They may not charge for work that is considered 'Category 1', i.e. work that is part of the normal NHS duties of hospital doctors. This includes:

1 the examination, diagnosis and furnishing of reports required in connection with treatment or prevention of an illness (paragraph 30 of the terms and conditions of service for hospital doctors)

2 furnishing reports on patients currently under treatment to the patient or a third party (including employers, the DSS and employment services) where it is reasonably incidental to treatment and does not involve substantial extra work

3 various other matters, for example mental health, court appearances etc listed in paragraph 36 of the terms and conditions of service for hospital doctors.

Hospital doctors may charge for so-called 'Category 2' work, which is described in paragraph 37 of the terms and conditions of service and includes:

1 examination of and reports on patients not under treatment

2 examination of and reports on patients who are under treatment but which involves an appreciable amount of extra work

3 examinations and reports requested by various authorities, government agencies, employers, insurance companies, solicitors etc

4 attendance at court (including the coroner's court)

5 mental health examination and reports at the behest of social services

6 other government work, medical boards, tribunals for the DSS/Benefits Agency etc.

All this work is so-called 'Category 2' work and is subject to the 'one-third' rule.[a] This requires that where laboratory, radiological or technical facilities

---

[a]Since 1994, NHS Trust hospitals have the right to impose their own level of charges for the use of NHS technical equipment, which may be more or less than one-third.

are used, doctors have to pay one-third of the gross fee to the hospital. These facilities do not include secretarial or administrative support. The 'one-third' rule does not apply to coroner's post mortems but does apply to other analytical work for coroners.

Charging for 'treatment'

GPs may not charge their own NHS patients for treatment. The interpretation of the word treatment is very wide and includes referral to specialists, whether NHS or private. Paragraph 38 of the terms of service (schedule 2 of the NHS General Medical Services Regulations 1992) lists the strictly limited circumstances in which GPs may charge fees to their NHS patients. The GP's NHS patients are defined in paragraph 4 of the terms of service. GPs contemplating making any charge to their NHS patients must ensure that they comply with the strict requirements of the terms of service and that they act in accordance with the ethical duty not to use, or appear to use, their position of trust to influence patients to follow a particular course of action that may offer the doctor some advantage, financial or otherwise. GPs must bear in mind that their action, in making a charge, could be alleged to involve accepting remuneration for treatment, which could be construed as breaching either their terms of service or their ethical duty not to abuse this position of trust. The consequences could be a complaint to the Family Health Services Authority (FHSA), with a possible finding of breach of the terms of service, a complaint to the General Medical Council's (GMC's) Professional Conduct Committee or, ultimately, criminal proceedings. GPs who are in any doubt about whether they may or may not charge a fee for something that may be construed as treatment should consult their local British Medical Association (BMA) office or their medical defence organisation.

How much to charge

Providing GPs meet the terms of their NHS contract, there is no limit to the amount that they may earn from private practice. However, if income from private work exceeds 10% of gross practice receipts, FHSA allowances for premises and staff used will be proportionately abated. This is covered in paragraph 52.19 of the Statement of Fees and Allowances (SFA).

Fees for almost all the services that GPs may provide privately are negotiated or considered by the Private Practice and Professional Fees

Committee of the BMA. This includes fees for local and central government departments, and reports and certificates for patients or third parties. The level of fees varies according to the work involved, but is largely calculated on a time-banded basis, except where it is governed by statute or represents the outcome of negotiations with a government department or other national body. Copies of the BMA guidance notes on fees for part-time medical services can be obtained by members of the BMA from their local offices.

For ease of reference, the fees are grouped into four broad categories, as given below.

Category A

These are fees prescribed by statute or statutory instrument, including fees for giving emergency treatment at road traffic accidents and certain specified work in connection with the Access to Medical Records Act and the Data Protection Act.

Category B

Category B comprises fees negotiated nationally (UK) with government departments and other employers. Until 1993, all government departments set their fees in line with the so-called 'Treasury general schedule'. This schedule was agreed between representatives of various government departments, including the Treasury, and representatives of the BMA in 1981. The agreement provided for annual uprating of the fees in line with the recommendations of the Doctors' and Dentists' Review Body (DDRB) and also for a triennial review of the baselines. Owing to refusal of the Treasury to take part, the triennial reviews never occurred, and in 1993 a new agreement was reached with the Treasury, which provided for a much shortened and simplified fee structure, together with significant increases in most of the fees. Although this new schedule was accepted by some government departments (e.g. the Driver and Vehicle Licensing Authority [DVLA], the Criminal Injuries Compensation Board and the Ministry of Defence), other government departments, such as the Department of Health (DoH), the Department of Social Security (DSS) and the Lord Chancellor's Department, all refused to implement the new Treasury schedule. Although some of them have applied a modest increase to the fee scales payable in 1993, the BMA has refused to agree these fees as providing a satisfactory level of remuneration, and there is no longer any national agreement between these government departments and the BMA on an appropriate scale of fees for providing the services that these departments request.

Category C

Category C covers fees negotiated nationally with other representative bodies. This includes fees for life assurance reports negotiated with the Association of British Insurers, and work for the provident associations and the ambulance associations. The agreement is binding only on members of the national body with whom the BMA has reached agreement, but in practice, it means that the agreed fees are paid in almost every case.

Category D

In Category D, there is fees guidance issued by the BMA for other private work. This includes fees not covered by negotiation or statute, i.e. those not included in the categories A to C described above. The level of fees is for agreement between the doctor and the party requesting the work. Where settlement of the fee is the responsibility of the patient or person to be examined, the level of the fee is a matter of mutual agreement, but the BMA issues guidance for its members on certain fees that are regarded as reasonable. In addition to those fees paid by the patient, this category also covers a wide variety of work for which no national agreement has been sought with representative bodies or on which no agreement can be reached. This now includes work for those government departments who have refused to implement the new Treasury scales.

The Private Practice and Professional Fees Committee (PPPFC) is elected annually by the Representative Body of the BMA and has two additional members appointed by the Council of the BMA. There are representatives from general practice, hospital medicine, community medicine and the Junior Doctors' Committee. The recommendations of the Committee concerning appropriate levels of fees and in connection with negotiated fees are submitted to Council for approval before they are published by the BMA.

Subsequent chapters in this book will go into more detail on the range of private services that GPs may provide for their NHS patients, and will also consider many of the sessionally paid opportunities for employment for doctors outside the NHS contract.

2   Work for central and local government

Frank McKenna

Local and central government continue to provide GPs with their largest supply of professional work outside the NHS. The exact nature of opportunities for GPs largely depends upon the commissioning body or agency. It mainly consists of providing factual reports on patients and carrying out medical examinations. Some work, for example GPs providing regular sessions for the Benefits Agency or local authorities, will be governed by contracts. It is important to ensure that the terms of these agreements or contracts are reasonable and that they offer an adequate level of remuneration. Given the extent of their NHS commitments, GPs should ensure that any time they have available to engage in private work is both clinically rewarding and financially attractive. Most GPs continue to underestimate the value their clinical skills can bring when working outside the NHS. Looking at other professions, such as lawyers and accountants, provides a useful comparator that should help GPs to estimate the value they place on their professional time.

The sections below offer general guidance to GPs who wish to increase their non-NHS earnings.

DSS/Benefits Agency Medical Services

The Benefits Agency Medical Services (BAMS), an executive agency of the DSS, provides some 70% of all central government work for GPs, varying from doctors employed on a regular part-time or sessional basis examining social security claimants who are ill or incapacitated, to individual GPs providing reports on their own patients. The introduction, in April 1995, of Incapacity Benefit (IB), which replaced Invalidity Benefit (IVB), is expected to increase dramatically the amount of medical information needed by BAMS to process social security claims in two significant ways. First, GPs will be required to give short factual statements to BAMS detailing the patient's main condition that prevents him from being employed. These certificates must be provided free of charge as they form a terms of service requirement for NHS GPs. Second, the number of sessional examinations

BAMS commissions each year will rise from 600 000 in 1994 to over 1.5 million in 1995 to take acount of the 'all work test', a new feature of IB assessment. Some 7000 doctors, mainly GPs, undertake regular sessional work for BAMS, examining claimants for benefits such as Attendance Allowance, Disability Living Allowance and IB.

Until 1993, fees for both part-time medical referees and item of service reports were agreed centrally between the BMA and the DSS/BAMS (see Chapter 1). However, these departments refused to implement an agreement between the Treasury and the BMA, and, as a result, there is no agreed level of remuneration for any work on behalf of BAMS. As a result, the BMA offered advice to its members suggesting that they either decline to perform these services until revised fees were agreed or, alternatively, charge their full market fees for these non-NHS services. While accepting that this amount of available work offered by BAMS is attractive for many practices, there is unlikely to be any radical improvement in part-time doctors' pay as long as GPs are prepared to work for unagreed levels of fees. GPs considering sessional work for BAMS should contact their local BMA office for advice on current suggested fees.

Driver and Vehicle Licensing Agency

The DVLA's medical branch commissions some 100 000 reports and examinations of drivers and prospective drivers each year, most of which are provided by GPs. In discharging its obligations to advise the Secretary of State for Transport on issuing driving licences, the DVLA is required by law to consider whether an applicant is fit to drive, i.e. whether the potential or current licence holder is suffering from a medical condition that materially affects his ability to drive safely.

Although there are certain prescribed disabilities that render a person unfit to drive, for example, epilepsy, severe mental disability or abnormal eyesight, there are other conditions, such as diabetes mellitus, poliomyelitis and muscle disease, that will need individual assessment to determine to what extent the applicant's ability to drive is affected. GPs may therefore, be asked to provide a report based either on a patient's notes or on a medical examination. This information will then be considered by the DVLA medical branch when deciding whether or not to issue or withdraw a driving licence. Unlike reports for insurance purposes, the DVLA does not ask GPs for an opinion on an individual's fitness to drive. The fees for medical reports, examinations and questionnaires were previously based on an agreement between the BMA and the DVLA. However, since 1995 no agreed fees have existed between the DVLA and the BMA and doctors have been advised to charge their market fees when performing this work. GPs who are BMA members may wish to contact their **local** BMA office for information on current suggested fees.

Apart from commissioning reports from an individual's GP, the DVLA also uses the services of around 150 doctors franchised to conduct independent examinations on individuals who, for example because of a court order, are required to undergo a separate medical examination before being reissued with a licence. Franchised doctors are generally selected from a list of local medical officers registered with the Civil Service Occupational Health and Safety Agency (OHSA), and are chosen geographically. Although their agreement to provide services is with the DVLA, licence applicants are liable for the doctor's professional fees. While this work is generally well paid, it is often sporadic and can, therefore, be a problematic source of income on which to rely.

Civil Service Occupational Health and Safety Agency

The Civil Service OHSA is responsible for promoting the health and safety of civil servants at work throughout central government departments and agencies. It also provides occupational health services to public bodies and other independent organizations. The OHSA's advice to clients is generally related to issues that have a bearing on decisions to be taken on the continuing employment or recruitment of a client's employee. As part of this process, GPs are often approached for information designed to enable a department to determine, for example, whether an employee's sickness record is *bona fide* or whether someone should be offered early retirement on medical grounds.

The OHSA requests over 25 000 reports each year from both hospital doctors and GPs. This work is in addition to that undertaken by the approximately 1000 local medical officers it retains throughout Great Britain to provide medical services, for example conducting an independent medical examination on employees. This work can be both clinically challenging and financially rewarding for GPs who are formally appointed to act as local medical officers.

Ministry of Defence

Many Ministry of Defence (MoD) establishments, for example military bases, rely heavily on surrounding GP practices to provide a range of supporting medical services, particularly locum cover. Although a large number of medical practitioners is directly employed through the armed services, i.e. the Royal Army Medical Corps personnel and civilian medical practitioners, the flexibility to purchase additional medical services as and when needed has become an increasingly attractive option for the MoD. GPs may be asked to provide a range of medical services to military bases including:

- locum cover to MoD establishments

- lectures on first aid

- release medicals

- immunisations and vaccinations (not covered by the NHS), with certificates

- large goods (LGV) and passenger carrying vehicle (PCV) examinations (including sight and hearing tests)

- maternity and contraceptive services.

The fees for this work were previously agreed centrally between the BMA and the MoD. However, since 1995, no agreement has existed, and GPs should, therefore, treat MoD bases as they would any private employer. BMA members can seek advice on current suggested fees from their **local** BMA office.

Collaborative Arrangements

As a result of health service reforms in 1974, the Secretary of State for Health delegated responsibility for the provision of public health, education and social services functions to health authorities and local authorities. These are commonly referred to as the 'Collaborative Arrangements'. GPs most frequently take on work under the Arrangements in relation to social service activities. These can range from being asked to examine an individual under the Mental Health Act to providing a report on a prospective childminder.

There is little opportunity to engage in regular sessional work under the Arrangements as most approaches to GPs are made on an item of service basis, in which only a particular medical report or opinion is needed for one of their patients. The fees for this work were previously agreed annually between the DoH and the BMA, but since 1994, no agreement has been reached, owing to the DoH's refusal to implement the fees recommended by the Treasury. This leaves GPs with two options: first, they can charge their full market rates for work under the Arrangements (the BMA's suggested fees for non-NHS services are a useful guide) and, second, they can decline to undertake work when asked by local authorities. Except for infectious disease notification (for which they can claim a fee), GPs are not obliged to provide any services to local or health authorities under the Arrangements. Most GPs will, however, in relation to the Mental Health Act, wish to assist patients by either making an examination or recommendation, regardless of the fee offered. In relation to individuals suffering from mental illness, GPs are entitled to claim a fee under the Mental Health Act for examining a patient, regardless of whether or not a recommendation to section is made. The fee, therefore, is payable because of the clinical examination, rather than the recommendation. The list below sets out some of the main services requested of GPs under the Arrangements. The types of services covered are:

- adoption and fostering reports and examinations for social service departments

- Mental Health Act assessments (and recommendations)

- examination of blind or partially sighted persons

- children in care proceedings – medical reports and examinations

- registration of prospective childminders (under the Children Act).

GPs who wish to find out more about the Collaborative Arrangements, and are BMA members, may wish to contact their **local** BMA office for advice and up-to-date information on suggested fees.

Doctors assisting local authorities

Although GPs are more commonly asked to provide services to local authorities under the Collaborative Arrangements, it is important not to overlook the other services that local authorities require and which can often provide a useful source of income. Work requested from GPs by local authorities differs from the Collaborative Arrangements on two counts. First, the services do not relate to the fields of education, public health or social services, and, second, the fees are directly reimbursed by the local authority, rather than the health authority. The fees, which are negotiated by the BMA with the Local Government Management Board through a joint negotiating committee, are revised each April and are generally in line with increases recommended by the Doctors' and Dentists' Review Body (DDRB).

BMA members can contact their **local** BMA office for a fees guidance schedule that sets out information on both the services provided by GPs and the current agreed level of fees. Listed below is a sample of the services offered by GPs to local authorities.

- Medical reports on local authority employees and prospective employees (including police officers and firefighters).

- Medical reports and examinations on local authority employees for superannuation purposes.

- Examinations for LGV and PCV drivers.

- General occupational health services.

- Medical referees to crematoria.

Much of this work is on an item of service basis and therefore available to all GPs, while other parts of it are usually undertaken on a sessional or contracted basis. The refusal of some government departments to implement an appropriate level of remuneration has made the work less attractive to many doctors, and GPs may wish to consider whether or not they really wish to undertake work for fees that are clearly below the market rate for the clinical skills and professional judgement they bring to these areas of work.

3   Private GP services

Geoffrey Samson

Private general practice gives the doctor the opportunity to provide personal high-quality primary medical and preventive health care without the involvement of a third party.

The private GP will need to provide premises, staff and equipment out of the income received by the practice. There will also be a need to make provision for sickness and retirement benefits from this source. These annual expenses can be expected to equal anything from 30 to 60% of the practice's gross income.

Private general practice is usually based on a personal contract between the patient and the doctor, the fees being based on an item of service basis, with a fixed fee for a consultation or a home visit. A few practices charge an annual subscription, with a smaller item of service fee and fees for child development checks or complete maternity care (excluding specialist fees should they be needed for maternity complications, for example caesarean section).

Some employers will pay the fees incurred by their employees with certain practices, and some foreign visitors and residents will have a private GP's fees reimbursed by their private health insurance.

The provident associations and insurance companies have, by and large, avoided involvement in primary health care insurance. This may be changing, and some companies are considering limited primary care insurance.

Advertising

The alteration of the rules on advertising by the GMC makes the setting up of a private practice easier, as there can now be direct advertising rather than a dependence on personal recommendation and word of mouth. The GMC has issued guidance on advertising medical services. Private general practices can provide the public with practice leaflets giving factual information about their qualifications, services and practice arrangements, and including a statement about their approach to medical practice. Up-to-date information of this kind should be available at doctors' consulting rooms. It may also be placed in libraries and other places where the public would normally expect to find information relating to their locality. Practices may distribute such information on an unsolicited basis within the areas they serve, providing no individual or group of patients is singled out to receive the information and that the distribution is not carried out in such a way as to put the recipients under pressure. GPs may also publish factual information on their services in the press, directories or other media. Doctors' services should not, however, be advertised by means of unsolicited visits or telephone calls with the aim of recruiting patients, as this would render the doctor liable to disciplinary proceedings by the GMC.

There is a general requirement that any advertising material must contain only that which is legal, decent, honest and truthful, and should conform with the other requirements of the British Code of Advertising Practice. In addition to those requirements, doctors publishing information about their services should not abuse the trust of patients or attempt to exploit their lack of medical knowledge. They must not offer guarantees to cure particular complaints. The material should contain only factual information and must not include any statement that could be regarded as misleading or, directly or by implication, as disparaging the services provided by other doctors. No claim of superiority should be made either for the services offered or for a particular doctor's personal qualities, qualifications, experience or skills.

Doctors are responsible for ensuring that any name plates, notice boards and other signs about their practices are sufficient to inform the public of the existence or location of the premises, while not being used to draw public attention to the services of one doctor or practice at the expense of others. In cases of doubt, it is advisable to consult one of the medical defence societies.

Various independent medical organisations now employ GPs and advertise medical services to the public. These include doctor visiting services, drop-in centres, which may provide consultations, health screening, vaccinations, counselling and pre-employment medicals etc, slimming clinics, private hospitals and nursing homes. The same advertising conditions apply, and the advertisements should not make invidious comparisons with the NHS or any other organisations or doctors, nor claim any superiority of the professional services offered or of any of the doctors connected with the organisation.

Doctors who have any kind of financial or professional relationship with such an organisation, or who use its facilities, are deemed by the GMC to bear some responsibility for the advertising, even if the doctor is unaware of the nature or content of the advertising and is unable to exert any influence over it. This applies to doctors who accept patients for examination or treatment who have been referred by such an organisation.

Doctors should also avoid promoting the services of such an organisation, for example by public speaking, broadcasting, writing articles or signing circulars. Doctors should neither permit the organisation's promotional material to claim superiority for their professional qualifications or experience, nor allow a personal address or telephone number to be used for enquiries on behalf of an organisation.

If a doctor is working for an organisation offering services directly to individual patients without reference from their own GP, the doctor has a duty to inform the GP immediately of any findings and recommendations before embarking on treatment, except in emergencies or unless the patient expressly withholds consent or has no regular GP. In such a case, the doctor must be responsible for the patient's subsequent care until another doctor has agreed to take over that responsibility.

Setting up in private practice

Although the easing of the rules on advertising by the GMC has made the setting up of private practice less hazardous, the general economic climate has not been conducive to this development, and there has been no large increase in the number of private practitioners, which remains at about 500 full-time private GPs. This is only a 'guesstimate' as there is no register of private practices. Private general practice tends to be concentrated in particular locations where there is a predominance of patients with high disposable incomes or of foreign residents, or where there are cultural factors at work.

The aspiring entrant to private general practice should remember the three 'As'.

1   **Affability:** A wide social circle and good bedside manner will attract and help to keep patients.

2   **Availability:** If a practitioner is to maintain a successful private practice, he or she will need to be readily accessible to give telephone advice or a consultation within a reasonable period of time, or be prepared to visit the patient as required. The practitioner is, however, under no legal obligation to provide these services unless he or she has made a specific

contract with the patient, unlike his or her NHS counterparts, who are bound by their terms of service.

3   **Ability:** The practitioner does not necessarily need to have any special qualifications, but it will often help to build up the practice if he or she has additional skills with experience in other fields.

Box 3.1: Useful additional degrees or diplomas

- MRCGP
- MRCP
- DCH
- DCROG
- Diploma in Sports Medicine
- Diploma in Physical Medicine
- MRCPsych.

Box 3.2: Useful additional skills

- psychotherapy
- homeopathy
- hypnosis
- acupuncture
- osteopathy/manipulative medicine.

Details of useful organisations for further training and postgraduate support are given at the end of the chapter.

Few private GPs earn more than NHS practitioners, and they tend to work longer hours for the same income. Most private GPs supplement their income by performing other medical services, such as company medicals and insurance work, part-time occupational health, travel clinics and sports medicine.

Some private GPs may be paid a retainer by a hotel or group of hotels, and are on call for the hotel patrons to whom they charge private fees.

NHS GPs are permitted to undertake any amount of private practice providing they fulfil their NHS commitments. However, if the GP uses premises or staff that are directly reimbursed for NHS purposes, and if the private practice income is more than 10% of the total practice receipts, these NHS reimbursements will be abated, so that if the private receipts are between 10 and 20% of the total receipts, an abatement of 10% is made on the NHS reimbursements; if the private receipts are between 20 and 30% of the total practice receipts, an abatement of 20% is made on the NHS reimbursements; and so on in 10% income bands.

Under their terms of service, NHS GPs are not allowed to charge a fee to their own or their partners' NHS patients, except for certain categories of fees.

An NHS GP cannot concurrently treat a patient both privately and on the NHS. GPs' terms of service prohibit them from accepting any payments from patients whose treatment they or their partners are responsible for under their NHS contract, unless payments are specifically authorised.

Some patients may choose to have both an NHS GP and a private GP from another practice. NHS GPs must only prescribe on NHS prescriptions (FP10) to their NHS patients; they cannot prescribe on NHS prescriptions for their private patients.

Box 3.3: Services for which a fee may be charged

- Holiday insurance certificate

- Blood test (not involving disputed paternity)

- Court of protection medical certificates

- Cervical cytology (non-NHS)

- Private medical consultations

- Copying medical notes

- Comprehensive medical examinations and reports

- Fitness to attend court as a witness

- Cremation forms B and C

- Removal of a pacemaker following death

- Pre-employment examinations

- Reports requested by employers

- Private sickness absence certificates for school or work

- Motor insurance certificates of fitness

- Accident and sickness insurance certificates

- Validation of provident association claim forms

- School fees insurance

- Fitness for higher education

- Fitness to participate in sport

- Freedom from infection certificate

- Vaccination and immunisation

- Attendances, at the patient's request, at police stations, that are not covered by an NHS fee

- Family planning

- Lecture fees

- Non-NHS minor surgery

- Seat belt exemption certificates

- Prescription for drugs required in overseas travel

- Reports for drug companies

- Race meetings and sporting activities

- Private nursing homes

- Data protection legislation: search of records

- Access to medical records: copying fee

- Reports on prospective subscribers to health insurance

- Non-medical services (e.g. passport signing)

- Payments to deputising doctors

- Fees for medico-legal work (i.e. professional witnesses and expert witnesses)

Fees guidance is available from the BMA for various types of private work.

Box 3.4: Services for which fees may not be charged

Death certificates

In England and Wales, the registered medical practitioner who was in attendance upon the deceased during his or her last illness must deliver a death certificate, stating to the best of his or her knowledge and belief, the cause of death to the local registrar forthwith, and he or she may not charge a fee for this service. Failure to deliver the certificate 'without reasonable excuse' is punishable on summary conviction with a fine. He or she must also hand the person designated as 'qualified informant' the outer detachable part of the certificate form entitled 'Notices to informant', duly completed.

Stillbirth certificates

Any registered medical practitioner who was present at the birth or examined the body of a stillborn child must, upon a request from the 'qualified informant', give a certificate stating that the child was not born alive, and, where possible, stating to the best of his or her knowledge and belief the cause of death and estimated duration of the pregnancy.

An NHS GP has unrestricted discretion as to whether to treat a non-EU visitor as an NHS patient or as a wholly private patient under the DoH circular HN(FP) (84) (7), apart from immediately necessary (i.e. emergency) treatment. The circular, however, also states that if no local NHS GP is willing to treat the non-EU visitor on an NHS basis, he or she can apply to the FHSA to be assigned to a local list of NHS GPs, in which case the GP to whom the patient is assigned is obliged to provide NHS service free of charge for the minimum number of days, as specified in the NHS terms of service.

Useful addresses

The British Post Graduate Medical
Foundation
33 Milner Street
London   WC1N

Tel: 0171–871 2222

Homeopathy
Royal London Homeopathic Hospital
Great Ormond Street
London   W1N

Tel: 0171–837 8833

British Homeopathic Association
27a Devonshire Street
London   W1N 1RJ

Tel: 071–935 2163

Acupuncture
British Medical Acupuncture Society
British College of Acupuncture
8 Hunter Street
London   WC1 BN

Tel: 0171–837 6429

Hypnosis
British Society of Medical and Dental
Hypnosis
Secretary:
42 Links Road
Ashtead
Surrey

Tel: 01372–273522

Psychotherapy
Centre for Counselling and Psychiatry
Education
21 Ladster Road
London   W11 1QL

Tel: 0171–221 3215

Osteopathy
British School of Osteopathy
1–4 Suffolk Street
London   SW1Y 4TG

Tel: 0171–930 9254

Independent Doctors Forum
President:
Dr F Clifford Rose
110 Harley Street
London   W1

Tel: 0171–935 3546

4 Opportunities in insurance work

Chris Evans and Spencer Leigh

Although a few doctors make a full-time living from insurance work, most GPs use it to supplement their NHS income, and an average GP may add £2000 per annum from this source to his salary.

The nature of the work

Most of the requests addressed to GPs concern life assurance benefits, for which medical information is required. These simple forms are called private medical attendant reports (PMARs). These request forms are similar for most companies, and an efficient, timely and professional response is sought and expected from GPs. The requests are for proposals for life assurance or, in the case of health insurance, at the point of claim, which may be on death or sickness. In either event, it cannot be stressed too strongly that the GP's prompt reply is essential.

Private medical attendant reports (PMARs)

PMARs do not require an examination and may be filled in quickly with reference to the patient's records. The standard fee is reviewed annually subject to agreement between the Association of British Insurers (ABI) and the BMA. Additional questionnaires, for example covering diabetes and, respiratory and cardiac conditions, attract extra monies according to their complexity. The usual PMAR includes simple questions on the person's medical history, and nowadays a computer printout listing present treatment and previous medical history may be accepted in lieu of the report.

Independent medical examinations (IMEs)

Medical examinations are carried out independently of the applicant's GP.

They are provided by consultant physicians and established GPs known to the life office. These also attract a fee that is subject to annual review. These independent medical reports are not subject to the legislation of the Access to Medical Reports Act 1988, and can be completed, signed, dated and returned promptly to the company.

Insurance companies are happy to add suitable doctors to these panels. Some use the services of professional medical services and examination companies to organise the examinations, which may be in the applicant's home. A list of useful addresses is to be found at the end of this chapter. Doctors may have to pay for inclusion on such a list, and may receive less than the agreed ABI/BMA fee for each examination, but the advantage is that many more examinations may be performed.

Relationship between doctor and insurance company and doctor and patient

The PMAR and the IME are always returned to the insurance company's chief medical officer. It would be impossible for the chief medical officer to handle all this mail, but the report is his responsibility and he delegates to staff who are permitted to review the information. Strict confidentiality is maintained in insurance companies, and GPs should have no fear about medical information having a general circulation. If the GP chooses to withhold information from the report, he should inform the insurance office that he has left out medical details in the patient's best interest (*see* below). Sometimes, applicants enquire of insurance companies the content of their medical report. GPs should be reassured that any enquiry about the PMAR between the insurance company and the applicant would only be made through the chief medical officer personally.

Doctor and patient

When the applicant fills in details of his own medical history in the proposal, he will also complete an authorisation for the release of details about his medical history to the insurance company. This authorisation has a standard text used by all insurance companies and follows the Access to Medical Reports Act 1988 (or equivalent legislation in Northern Ireland). Under this legislation, the applicant is entitled to see the report before it is returned to the insurance company. In practice, only 3–4% of applicants take up their right. If the right has not been exercised within 21 days, the GP can forward the report to the insurance company. When the applicant sees the report, he may comment on anything that has been written down, and he can request that certain information is not passed on to the insurance company. Similarly, the GP may omit certain information from the report if he considers it is not in the patient's interest to see it. After viewing, the GP should return the report to the insurance company with a note if he has not been in a position to complete it. The insurance company will recognise this position and still pay the fee.

Even when an applicant has indicated that he does not want to see his report, he is still entitled to see it for up to six months thereafter. Thus, GPs should keep a copy of the medical report and, under legislation, are entitled to charge a 'reasonable fee', paid by the applicant, for accessing the report.

Types of insurance for which medical information is required

Most requests for medical information will relate to life assurance benefits. For a regular monthly premium, an applicant is able to obtain insurance cover payable at a future age or on death. For example, a young fit applicant may pay £20 per month to obtain £200 000 life assurance. The benefit may be payable on death or on terminal illness, when the payout in full may be paid in advance if the policy holder has been told that he has less than 12 months to live.

A new form of insurance pays out the benefits if the policy holder develops certain nominated critical illnesses, such as a myocardial infarction or a life-threatening cancer. A popular form of insurance in the UK is permanent health insurance (PHI), in which a sickness benefit is paid if the applicant is away from work for perhaps six months or more.

Other insurance policies may pay hospital expenses or, in a recent development, meet the bills for long-term care.

Insurance companies endeavour to offer cover to their applicants, and many people with even serious medical impairments will be offered policies. Indeed, more than 95% of all insurance proposals are accepted at standard rates of premium. About 4% of applicants will be charged an extra premium because of health problems, and the remainder will be declined or deferred, either because of the medical history or because they are awaiting investigation or treatment.

What are insurance companies seeking?

Life assurance

It is not economic for an insurance company to obtain a medical report for every application received. About 60% of proposals for life insurance are accepted without any independent medical corroborative evidence. The companies are taking a calculated risk with their proposers, since some applicants may be economical with the truth when they fill in details of their own medical state. Nevertheless, insurance companies have limits based on the sum assured at which they automatically request medical evidence. These limits differ from company to company and increase with inflation. Typical levels (1995) are given in Table 4.1.

Table 4.1 Typical levels (1995) based on sum assured

	Sum assured (£)	
Age of applicant	PMAR	IME
Less than 40	100 000	200 000
41–50	60 000	120 000
51–60	30 000	60 000
61–65	15 000	30 000
Over 65	5 000	10 000

An office will request a PMAR below this level if adverse features are revealed in the applicant's proposal. For example, a PMAR will be requested if there is a history of depression, but a PMAR and IME will be obtained if the applicant reveals he is an insulin-dependent diabetic. The PMAR requests details of:

- previous illnesses, hospital consultations and hospital admissions
- current medical treatment
- specific questions regarding sexually transmitted diseases, mental illness and intemperance
- any known blood pressure readings, urine analysis, or other investigations.

In particular, insurance companies wish to know about aspects of the family history, for example familial polyposis coli, Huntington's chorea or polycystic kidneys, that might actually affect life expectancy. They will expect to be informed about the results of health checks, such as for cholesterol and uric acid levels, liver function tests and blood count, and random blood glucose readings, especially those tests in the private sector about which they have details. Any previous episode suggestive of premature vascular disease, such as angina, claudication or a transient ischaemic attack, would be important to mention.

While there is no need to include trivial illnesses such as coryza, a history of low back pain, while of little significance in assessing a life assurance proposal, may be all important for sickness insurance (see below).

The IME is a much more comprehensive form of assessment. It consists of:

- a health questionnaire

- details of medical and family history

- life-style questions

- measurement of height, weight, blood pressure, urine analysis, chest expansion, abdominal girth and possibly peak expiratory flow rate

- examination of the whole applicant, including heart, lungs, abdomen, central nervous system, joints, glands and skin.

GPs should note that, before commencing the IME, one should carefully read the instructions of the company and, if possible, have sight of the PMAR, so that one's clinical skills are directed to the particular relevant aspect.

While the medical assessment of the proposal lies with the chief medical officer of the company, the doctors performing the IME may be asked to categorise the applicant as standard, impaired or unacceptable. In addition, if the applicant is undergoing investigation and treatment for which there are insufficient medical details, the recommendation should be for a deferral while relevant reports are obtained. There will be occasions when, for example, a heart murmur is discovered and one is unsure of its significance. In these circumstances the finding should be fully described and, if indicated, further assessment (e.g. echocardiography) requested. If the history and examination indicate that an ECG is required, for example with a history of a previous myocardial infarction or current angina, the ECG should be performed, for which a fee should be agreed by the GP in advance. The detection of glycosuria, albuminuria and haematuria can never be ignored and require further assessment. If crackles that do not clear on coughing are heard in the chest, a chest X-ray is mandatory, and ultrasound examination of the abdomen should be recommended for any palpable mass.

Sickness claims

An insurance company will want clinical evidence when it is asked to pay out sickness benefits, which could be a lump sum under a critical illness policy or regular monthly payments up to normal retirement age under a sickness policy. The GP may be asked to provide details of the claimant's illness and provide medical reports. A GP performing an IME under such a policy may be asked to conduct an examination of a claimant who is not his patient. There are currently no agreed fees for this work between the BMA and ABI.

Early death claims

Insurance companies repudiate very few death claims, despite newspaper articles to the contrary. Insurance claims are frequently paid when death is by suicide or as a result of AIDS. The principal area of discussion is when death occurs in the first two years after the policy has been effected. If a PMAR was originally obtained, no problems should arise, but if the proposal was accepted on the applicant's evidence alone, the office may wish to check whether fraud or non-disclosure had occurred. In such circumstances, a GP may be sent a so called 'duration certificate', seeking answers to questions about the patient's last illness. A fee is due for this service, which is a matter for individual consideration.[a]

What should GPs disclose to patients?

Most IME forms ask the GP not to reveal the findings to the applicant. However if one were, for example, to find a breast lump or significant hypertension, it would be the GP's duty to encourage applicants to seek urgent attention from their own GP. Conversely, there is no requirement to inform the applicant that one considers his application substandard and potentially loadable, as insurance companies differ in their assessment of

[a]Editor's note: The BMA's ethical advice is that the duty of confidentiality extends beyond death. The BMA advises doctors, as a general rule, not to release information to insurance companies about a deceased patient unless the provisions of the Access to Health Records Act apply. GPs also have the duty to withhold information of sensitive nature which they believe the deceased patient would have wished to remain confidential. GPs may seek written advice on these issues from the BMA's Medical Ethics Committee.

medical risks and impairment, and some types of contract – for example a young patient with an endowment proposal compared with an elderly patient with term assurance – are able to accommodate medical impairment more than others.

As the applicant's GP, one is entitled to contact the company's chief medical officer, who will be happy to discuss how a particular proposal has been assessed.

HIV testing

Most offices have limits above which they request HIV testing automatically. Currently (1995) these are:

- single men – £150 000

- married men, and women – £250 000.

If there is a perceived risk factor, such as hepatitis B infection, sexually transmitted disease, haemophilia requiring factor VIII replacement or drug abuse, the applicant may be asked to attend for an HIV test, even for levels below those given above. When the test is included with the medical examination, there is usually an additional fee, a higher additional fee being offered if the test is requested in isolation from the examination. The insurance company will send the GP a kit for blood testing. It is necessary to provide counselling before the sample is taken, and the applicant must be made aware of the possible consequences of a positive result. The GP must ask the applicant to nominate a doctor who, in the event of the test proving positive, will arrange appropriate counselling. As there are no agreed fees between the BMA and the insurance industry for HIV testing, GP's are advised to seek advice from their **local** BMA office before agreeing to undertake this work.

Gaining entry to panels of examiners

GPs wishing to do more insurance work than merely PMARs on their own patients have several options. They can make contact with insurance offices, for whom they can perform PMARs, or they can contact some of the national organisations arranging IMEs on behalf of life offices. Most of these organisations reimburse GP's below the agreed ABI/BMA rate as BMA suggested fees for professional work. GP's must bear this in mind when considering these positions.

In submitting an application to a life office or national examination organisation, GPs should be prepared to give the following information.

1   Address and telephone and, if applicable, fax and mobile telephone numbers.

2   The names and qualifications of the medical members available in the practice to perform insurance examinations, and whether or not any are female.

3   Whether the practice members are willing or able to perform HIV testing, ECGs, exercise ECGs, chest radiography and urine microscopy.

4   What the availability for consultations for insurance examinations is – for example every weekday, Saturday morning or Tuesday afternoon only.

5   Whether a female chaparone will attend if required.

6   Whether a practice member is willing to do domiciliary visits.

Some insurance companies may seek from GPs a PMAR in respect of motor insurance. GPs may also charge their patients for filling in and providing medical evidence for the completion of personal or corporate claim forms dealing with private consultations with specialists.

Warning

Although the quality of GP reports and examinations is rarely in doubt, the speed at which they are completed and returned to the insurance company can sometimes be slow. Insurance companies compete with each other on service, and a recent development has been the introduction of paramedicals, whereby a shortened medical examination is performed in the applicant's home by an SRN. An insurance company may use this to replace either a GPs report or an IME. This is a threat to GPs' work, and its use may grow. It is therefore important that PMARs and IMEs are returned promptly. After all, the applicant wishes to be covered as soon as possible, so this is only fair to him, too.

Finally, for those who find insurance medicine fascinating, especially as much of its work involves the leading edges of modern medicine, such as HIV testing and genetic fingerprinting, much valuable information can be gleaned through membership of the Assurance Medical Society. Even if one cannot attend their meetings, their published proceedings are invaluable.

Useful addresses

Association of British Insurers (ABI)
51 Gresham Street
London   EC2V 7HQ

Tel: 0171–600 3333
Fax: 0171–696 8999

Assurance Medical Society
Lettsom House
11 Chandos Street
London   W1 0EB

Tel: 0171–636 6308
Fax: 0171–580 5793

Insurance Medical Services
15 Barbican Mews
London   W6 7PA

Tel: 0171–603 4598
Fax: 0171–603 4612

Medicals Direct
72 Shipston Road
Stratford Upon Avon
Warwickshire   CV37 7LR

Tel: (01789) 204079

National Medical Examination Network
Definitech
15–23 Tentercroft Street
Lincoln   LN5 7DB

Tel: (01522) 513450
Fax: (01522) 513458

UK Underwriting Services
Barclay's House
51 Bistopril
Horsham
West Sussex   RH12 1QJ

Tel: (01403) 217222
Fax: (01403) 217444

5 Working as a locum or deputy in general practice

Adrian Midgley

GPs are likely to become full-time locums at two points in their career – before entering GP partnership as a Principal and after NHS retirement. Each time it is a larger change than is either entering training or becoming a partner. Finishing vocational training, or retiring from a partnership, means leaving a secure organisation to become proprietor of a small business. Careful attention and planning reduces personal stress and increases profits.

Opportunities and income

Imposing the 1990 GP contract caused a demographic whiplash with a brief surplus of doctors available to work as locums, followed by the present moderate but persistent shortage. With an increased work-load in general practice and less tolerance of a delay in seeing a GP, there is more demand for locums. At the same time, there are pressures to increase the standard of care.

More vocationally trained doctors are choosing to avoid permanent practice and continue as long-term locums. Approached seriously and carefully, it is possible to make a satisfactory living from it. It can also avoid some of the more peculiar enthusiasms of the DoH and allow great flexibility in working practice.

There are no fixed rates for locums. The guidance prepared by the Private Practice and Professional Fees Committee of the BMA is just that; it forms a starting point from which to work. Local guidelines circulated to practices by groups of locums have more force and, of course, tend closely to resemble the BMA guidance. The BMA's suggested rates for deputies are rarely achieved in practice.

Preparation

Before you start your business, **prepare** a business plan, even if this only consists of working as much as you can for whatever deputising companies/ GP practices offer. Take as an example the idea that, as a fully trained GP, you now hope to earn a little more than you did in your trainee year, or that, as a very experienced GP, you expect to make as much as the junior partner replacing you. Add to this the expenses you propose to list on your tax return, and divide by the amount of work you are prepared to do. This is your target price per hour. Now repeat the exercise for the minimum you can support your standard of living on. This is your lowest acceptable rate.

You then enter **negotiations** knowing what the personal consequences of your agreement will be, and, if you find that you are accepting lower figures, you know that you must act in an organised fashion to change the rates, your life-style or both. As a general principle, do not accept jobs that do not pay your selected minimum rate. Unless you reduce your targets, you would be resentful in such jobs, which is unlikely to benefit anyone.

It is essential to agree the basis on which you will charge before you do the job. This may vary. For instance, you might agree to be on call after a surgery for the practice you live next to, sitting at home in the daytime for a modest fee, whereas travelling many miles to another practice and staying there would reasonably be paid at a higher rate. Some locums prefer to agree rates for surgeries and visits separately, but there is merit in charging by the hour as with many other professional groups, and adding mileage. The trend is towards simplification, with an hourly rate regardless of the nature of the work. This is helpful to practices who can buy the cover they need.

Deputising

Deputising is less of a wrench than becoming a locum. Deputising agencies are organised to different degrees, varying between the extremes of shambolic and oppressive. The same applies to the work.

Deputising sessions are hard work, not well paid and unlikely to lead to great personal satisfaction. However, they do provide an income, and the reduction of stress produced by a 'dispatcher' and a driver, compared with doing the same work on one's own, should not be underestimated. Being driven around an area may give you a clear idea of where you would or would not like to work and introduce you to the local practices.

A long-term contract as a deputy is a more appetizing prospect, with a salary of the order of the net mean intended annual remuneration for work that is sufficient to keep you, while allowing an occasional locum session at a prospective practice to keep up other interests. As a way of getting to know an area and meeting or becoming known to local principals, it is worth considering.

Deputising is, of necessity, subject to closer surveillance than most medical practice, so you should allow a lead time of at least two months to make arrangements before you need the work.

Requirements before deputising are:

- an interview with the medical representative of the deputising service

- references to be taken up

- your registration by the deputising service, as a deputy.

Circumstances that can make life miserable for locums are:

- five-minute bookings in an appointment surgery

- being booked for one surgery a day, but finding that another surgery has been cancelled and you are swamped with acute cases and extras

- an excessive number of visits (more than 4) per session

- a large practice area

- difficult traffic conditions

- poor signposting of streets and a lack of house names or numbers

- a practice with low morale (more common recently)

- an inefficiently run practice where you dislike working

- a computer that defies all logic and is provided with no basic instructions

- bad handwriting and disorganised notes

- being too reticent to charge your proper fees.

Agencies

If you are reasonably well organised, the value of someone else booking and billing your work should be no more than £5 per job. Agencies look for more than this, since they do not wish to charge much more than locums who organise their work directly with practices. If you join in with this, you are effectively competing against yourself. Having decided on a rate, this should be the income you look for whoever is paying the bill.

Locum groups

For many reasons, it is an excellent idea to join a group of practitioners with similar interests in your area. Small groups from vocational training schemes may continue, but more usually there will be a group of locums who form something between a trade association and a support group. If one cannot be found, you should start one.

Locum groups may become more important when accreditation of locums is clarified as one of the criteria for accreditation should be membership of a peer group within which to continue medical education and audit or quality control. Educational credits for locums and deputies will inevitably be similar to PGEA, and locum groups already organise PGEA-accredited meetings.

Locum groups are not agencies and should not take responsibility for their members.

Functions of a non-principal group

- To improve the life of GPs working other than as principals.

- To minimise inconsistencies in pay and reduce exploitation of locums, deputies and assistants, by agreeing and publicising consensus views.

- To provide a forum for discussion and mutual support.

- To assist members and local principals in organising locum work.

- To encourage and provide a framework for members' continuing education.

- To share information on administration, personal finance and job opportunities.

- To make representations to the BMA and other medical and statutory organisations on behalf of members, and locums in general, and to channel communications back to members.

Composition and constitution of a locum support group

Simply put, it is your group and its format is up to you, the members. There is a wide range of organisations on which you can model a group, ranging from the sybaritic medical dining club described in *How to do it*, to the 'sit in a circle' RCGP/vocational training scheme model. Below are some suggestions.

Officers

Since the officers are more likely to attend meetings, you may wish to have as many as you can think of a title for, but experience shows that you need three, who are:

- the treasurer
- the secretary
- the chairperson.

A meeting co-ordinator or organiser, a press officer and a negotiator need not, but could be, separate people.

Duties of the officers

The treasurer is responsible for acquiring, concentrating and accounting for funds, and disbursing small sums as expenses to cover the work of the group on behalf of its members. A formal constitution, naming the bankers and identifying those who may sign cheques (ideally two signatories for each cheque) should be drawn up.

The secretary is responsible for maintaining a list of all members, with up-to-date addresses and telephone numbers, circulating this list to local general practices and members at suitable intervals, and promulgating the details of meetings.

The chairman is responsible for conducting meetings, and arranging with the other officers and members where and when these will be.

Requirements and qualifications of the officers

- The treasurer should be honest and able to add up!
- The secretary should be mildly obsessional and must be the owner of a computer and a decent printer.
- The chairperson should enjoy the confidence of the members and be willing to find out what they want from the group. They could arrange for pharmaceutical representatives to provide support, in accordance with the code of practice published by the ABPI.

The best candidates for all three offices are those doctors who are likely to remain in the area for some time, such as doctors on the Retainer Scheme.

Conduct of the group's business

The group should meet regularly. Few organisations meet in August, but medical training is arranged so as to produce large numbers of newly trained GPs on 31 July each year. Invite them to the June meeting, or hold an August meeting; few locums should be on holiday in August. An adequate number of meetings should be arranged each year to deal with all relevant business matters and to provide time for continuing education.

Formal talks from consultants or other experts are best held in suitable rooms, whether in a postgraduate centre or a meeting room of a hotel or pub. Business meetings always work best in a member's home and should be rotated round the members and the geographic area.

Meetings should start – and end – on time.

Representing your locum support group

Your group should maintain contact with and make representations to:

- the BMA Private Practice and Professional Fees Committee
- the Locum Accreditation Working Party of the GMSC
- the FHSA
- the local medical committee
- the regional adviser in general practice.

These will generally be annual tasks, ranging from briefly discussing matters and sending a letter, to sending a representative to meetings.

- Co-ordinate your efforts with representatives of the other locum groups.
- Turn up on time for meetings (i.e. five minutes before the advertised starting time).
- Dress for meetings appropriately, eg suit jacket and tie.
- Concentrate on the most important things.
- Take notes.
- Pass on a briefing to your successor.

Representation

Representation of locums and deputies nationally is through the Locums and Deputies Working Party of the BMA's Private Practice and Professional Fees Committee. This working group reports to its parent committee and primarily addresses issues relating to locum rates.

Locum groups have provided representatives and written evidence to the working party of this committee and the GMSC in previous years, and other groups should aim to do likewise. The BMA needs to avoid appearing to act as a cartel of employers, and therefore pays genuine attention to representing them.

Locally, the LMC should represent your interests, but this cannot happen unless they know what these needs are. It is possible for the LMC to co-opt members to represent interests not already represented. This might offer an entry to medical politics for those who wish it.

Training

There are no specific qualifications or training programmes for locums or deputies. This is probably as it should be, since what the locum does is general practice – nothing else. Effective locums are conversant with the computer systems used in the practices in which they work. To ignore these risks missing vital information, to a patient's detriment, and generates extra work for the practice staff and doctors who see the patients later.

Vocational training schemes should recognize the particular characteristics of what is the next job for 80% of trainees. If you lecture to the vocational training scheme as an established locum, it is worth a fee.

Technology

Depending on the sort of work you do, and your home arrangements, you may find various technological devices useful. The foremost is the telephone answering machine, and you should make it a point of honour to answer all messages. Even if you cannot do that job, another will probably have arisen since the message was left.

The mobile phone is enormously useful, more so than a pager.

Given a computer for any other reason, it is sensible to keep your accounts on a spreadsheet. Faxing notes to practices from it may also avoid rushing around the following morning.

Conclusion

Locum and deputising work can be varied and satisfying, and providing you are well organised and come to sensible, clear arrangements with deputising services and employing practices, it can provide a satisfactory level of income. It allows locums and deputies the maximum flexibility to organise both professional and domestic commitments, free from the financial burden of being a principal, and free from the responsibilities of organising and running a practice.

6 Police surgeon (forensic medical examiner) work

Hugh de la Haye Davies

How to become a police surgeon

There are 43 police forces in England and Wales, seven police forces in Scotland and the Royal Ulster Constabulary in Northern Ireland.

The BMA, in agreement with local authorities and the Home Office, suggests, as a guideline, that one police surgeon and one deputy police surgeon be appointed per 100 000 population, but because of the different requirements of the 51 different police forces this figure is adapted to local conditions.

The larger forces, such as the Metropolitan Police (where, incidentally, police surgeons are called forensic medical examiners), have no difficulty in finding doctors of the right calibre who are willing to undertake the necessary training, as the individual case-load results in a substantial income. At the other extreme, doctors in less populated areas find that the low case-load, and subsequently low income, is not worth their being reasonably available at all times to answer police calls, with their more important practice commitments also needing attention. In these areas, the police have to rely on local practices doing the work on an *ad hoc* basis, which is an unsatisfactory situation, as there is no one doctor the police can rely on to carry out the forensic work, and there is also little financial incentive to undergo the necessary training in clinical forensic medicine.

The most common method of appointing police surgeons used to be from one particular practice, the position being taken on by succeeding partners as the senior partner retired. However, in these days of larger practices, it is not uncommon for the majority of partners in a practice not to wish to undertake the work, and those who do, feel they do not wish to put their hard earned, mostly nocturnal, earnings into the practice pool.

Therefore, many doctors who may be interested are dissuaded. More enlightened practices have an arrangement whereby the availability fees and day-time item of service fees are paid into the practice, but night-time fees are kept by the individual doctor and not put into the practice pool. If several partners in a practice are all doing police work, it makes sense that all earnings are paid into the common pool. With larger practices doing the work, this system is satisfactory from the partnership point of view but not good for the police, as the forensic work is diluted, with possibly no one doctor getting enough forensic experience. It often happens in such set-ups that when a serious forensic case occurs, the junior partner (or even the trainee) is on duty for the practice rota and, by custom, also on duty for the police. Many forces, even those with difficulty in recruiting police surgeons, do not like paying an availability fee (previously known as a retainer fee) to a practice, but would rather stipulate a named doctor and a named deputy. This is the basis of the national agreement negotiated by the BMA with the local authorities. The Association of Police Surgeons (APS) also supports this view, as it should mean that the police are able to call a forensically trained doctor when necessary.

The best way to find out about local arrangements is to ask the local police surgeon if he would like some help, especially at holiday times or weekends. This, at least, would give an insight into the work, and having carried out such non-retained duties may be a useful asset if one later applies for a position as a police surgeon or deputy. Unfortunately, being private practice, it is a fact of life that many appointed police surgeons are reluctant to allow other colleagues 'into their patch', although not all are of this disposition, and there are, especially in the ranks of the APS, many who are enthusiastic about their work who are also willing to impart their knowledge and expertise to younger colleagues. Local police superintendents or chief inspectors are also a useful source of information on prospects in their local area. Some doctors making even tentative enquiries find themselves being instantly persuaded to fill a vacuum that especially in some of the less populated areas has existed for a very long time.

Enquiries may also be made to the Secretary of the APS, who is often asked by police forces to assist in finding suitable doctors to fill vacancies in their force's area. Some forces place advertisements in the medical and lay press (especially the *British Medical Journal* classified section), but the majority of vacancies are made known by word of mouth. Selection procedures vary countrywide, the larger forces having a proper appointments panel with considerable medical input, usually from one or two senior police surgeons, but other forces, especially in less populated areas, being so glad to find someone that an offer of help is eagerly taken advantage of. Useful addresses are given at the end of the chapter.

Police surgeon work is not for the faint hearted. Both literally and metaphorically, it covers a multitude of sins. Fifty per cent of the work occurs between the hours of midnight and 8 am. Also, medical opinions are subject to cross-examination in any court of the realm, from the local magistrates to crown courts. The work, although hard, is extremely interesting; like any other job, it has its dull moments, but there are, more often than not, periods of excitement and intense activity. When one leaves the house or surgery to answer a call, one never knows what the end result will be. The uncertainty and variety of the work are fascinating, but above all the excellent relationships one develops with all ranks of the force, who are so appreciative of everything done for them, more than compensates for the irregular hours. Job satisfaction is high – at the end of the day it is worth while not only if you have made a contribution to bringing some villain to a guilty verdict, but equally so if at an early stage in police enquiries, you are able to help prevent innocent people being wrongly accused and sometimes even families being destroyed (this latter scenario being especially true with child abuse cases in some parts of the UK).

The nature of the work

Broadly speaking, the work can be divided into non-forensic and forensic duties. Non-forensic work may be loosely described as general practice in a police station setting – because of certain constraints, the prisoner, or maybe victim of crime, is unable to visit the surgery. Although it can be described largely as general practice, there are certain points of difference to bear in mind, the main one being that, in practice, the patient usually tells his GP the truth. In police surgeon work, the client (prisoner, victim or even policeman) may only tell the doctor what he thinks will help his case. A high degree of suspicion is necessary for the job – the approach is more 'veterinary' than medical. It is useful to examine the injuries first and then ask oneself, 'Are my findings consistent with what I have been told?' If not, one's index of suspicion becomes even more raised.

Non-forensic work includes people who are genuinely ill, and quite often a decision must be made on whether or not the person is fit to be detained, remembering that many conditions that can be safely treated at home (e.g. more than mild infections, fever, the later stages of pregnancy, some complications of diabetes and neurological cases) are not suitable for detention in the cold comfort of a police cell. In such cases, alternative arrangements must be made, the prisoner either being released on police bail or, if it is possible, sent to a prison hospital wing (as the illness is often not severe enough for admission to an NHS hospital).

Fitness to be interviewed often has to be assessed, and although ideally many cases would be helped by a psychiatric opinion, time and other constraints mean that this is not, in reality, possible. A good common-sense GP assessment carried out before, and if necessary after, interview will withstand most cross-examinations. Care of drug addicts in police custody is a specialty in itself. A full and proper examination after the taking of an (alleged) history should enable the doctor to keep the patient in reasonable comfort during his period of detention and also fit for interview, without giving in to his invariably excessive demands.

Taking blood samples under the Road Traffic Act is not such a common procedure these days as it was prior to the use of evidential breath machines in police stations, but on some occasions (usually of machine failure), the doctor is called in. In most cases, when a doctor is called for Road Traffic Act cases, it is to perform a comprehensive examination to decide whether the person is fit or 'unfit for the time being to have proper control of a motor vehicle due to being under the influence of drink or drugs'.

The forensic component of the work includes the initial examination of a dead body 'to confirm for police purposes that there is no *prima facie* evidence of foul play'. If there is any suspicion, a Home Office pathologist will attend, but there may be some tasks to be undertaken before their arrival. Generally speaking, minimum interference with the scene means no further action until their arrival. In some areas, many scenes are not visited by the pathologist, especially now that videorecording can produce an accurate record of the activities of the scene of crime team (including demonstration of the police surgeon's mistakes!).

The greater majority of the forensic work includes examination of victims in rape cases, woundings and other crimes against the person, and also the taking of samples (hair, blood, saliva, trace evidence etc). The alleged perpetrators of the crimes are usually also examined and samples collected. Accurate notes and well-composed reports are an essential sequel to these examinations, and the doctor may well later have to attend court, possibly being cross-examined on their work and opinion.

Box 6.1: Forensic and non-forensic duties

Forensic duties

- Examination in volent, unnatural and suspicious deaths – accidents, suicide, murder and deaths most commonly natural but in suspicious circumstances

- Examination of victims and assailants in crimes against the person – assaults, wounding, sexual offences and child abuse cases

- The taking of forensic samples, packaging them and arranging their secure storage and transport to the forensic laboratory

Non-forensic duties

- Examining prisoners with health problems

- Certifying fit for detention

- Certifying fit for interview

- Mental health assessments/recommendations

- Taking blood samples for Road Traffic Act cases

- Care of substance misusers in custody

- Examining prisoners alleging police assault

- Examining injured police officers

Although these duties are termed non-forensic and attract a lower item of service fee, there may be considerable medico-legal implications, emphasizing the need for properly trained police surgeons to deal with both forensic and non-forensic cases.

Contracts

Most police forces now have contracts with their doctors, based on the national agreement between the BMA and Local Authorities, which is reviewed annually. The fees are, in general, increased by the percentage that the government applies to NHS doctors after the annual DDRB report.

Discussions with the Local Authorities are currently taking place that may remove certain anomalies and, especially for rural doctors, enable GPs to be paid on a time basis, as recommended by the BMA for non-NHS work. (Current rates available to BMA members can be obtained via local BMA offices.) Holders of the Diploma in Medical Jurisprudence (DMJ) are recognized as specialists in clinical forensic medicine by the police forces.

There is a basic availability fee (formerly called a retaining fee) to compensate the doctor for having to make special arrangements to be 'reasonably available' to attend promptly police calls. This does not necessarily mean that everything has to be dropped and the doctor turn out immediately (as apart from blood alcohol cases, this is not necessary), but that after proper communication and discussion with the appropriate police officer, a mutually agreed time can be decided that is reasonable to both parties. It must be stressed that although most police calls are not medically urgent, a reasonably prompt attendance is indicated for police and legal purposes. It is not good enough if a prisoner is waiting for interview under the Police and Criminal Evidence Act to wait three hours to finish a surgery before examining him to see whether or not he is fit to be interviewed, as this may seriously prejudice police enquiries now that prisoners must be charged or released after certain time limits. A prisoner alleging violence perpetrated by the police is again better seen as soon as possible, for the sake of both parties.

Apart from the basic availability fees, with a supplement for DMJ holders or those longer than 15 years in post, there are item of service fees, depending on the type of case, on the time the service is rendered and on whether or not a statement is provided. Figure 6.1 summarises current fees in July 1995.

Figure 6.1: Fees for police surgeons/forensic medical examiners

Day cases (between 8 am and 7 pm)

Forensic	1st case	£40.80
(higher fee)	2nd and subsequent cases	£27.20
Non-forensic cases	1st case	£30.00
(lower fee)	2nd and subsequent cases	£20.00

Time taken over 1 hour, £26.50 per hour or part thereof

Night work (between 7 pm and 8 am)

Forensic	1st case	£61.20
	2nd and subsequent cases	£40.80
Non-forensic cases	1st case	£45.00
	2nd and subsequent cases	£30.00

Time taken over 1 hour, £40.80 per hour or part thereof.

Reports £24.30
Examinations of recruits £27.80
Police surgeon availability fee £2310 per annum
Deputy police surgeon £450 per annum
Supplementary payment (holders of DMJ) £780.00

Training

With increasing knowledge and sophistication of techniques used by criminals, and with the improved and more sophisticated methods of crime detection, especially in the forensic science field, it is essential that any doctor employed for this work is well trained. A one-week residential course is available for police surgeons prior to appointment, or within one year of appointment, at the National Training Centre for Scientific Support to Crime Investigation, a department of the Durham Constabulary. Most police forces send their 'novice' police surgeons, and, by arrangement with the Postgraduate Training Scheme, the course is recognised as six days for PGEA purposes. Experienced police surgeons, forensic scientists and police officers contribute to the course, at the end of which the students take part in a courts exercise, in which they are cross-examined by real solicitors on a case they have worked on during the week. 'Survivors' tell me that they found this an excellent preparation for their first court appearance. Quite a few have even said the 'Durham experience is worse than the real thing'! Certainly, those I have observed giving evidence have acquitted themselves well and obviously benefited from their training.

The Association of Chief Police Officers has recognised the value of this introductory course and have now an official policy that regular development courses should also be run every three or four years for established police surgeons. Although a Regional Development Course is run each year at Durham (in addition to the two or three initial training courses), each police region is responsible for the organisation of a series of half-day or weekend courses to cover all the modules in the development course syllabus. This gives doctors an opportunity to keep up to date in the manner best suited to their personal circumstances. For example, a doctor in Cumbria who does not wish to attend his own regional course (½ day a week for 12 weeks in Manchester) could go on a residential course in Durham for a week, or elsewhere for three weekends. All tastes are catered for, so there is no excuse for doctors to say there are now no training facilities to enable them to keep up to date.

The APS has been the progenitor of all these advances in training, and its senior members have an input into other training courses held at universities, postgraduate centres and forensic science laboratories all over the UK. The APS itself has an annual conference for three days in May and an autumn symposium for two days in September; Metropolitan Group holds a January meeting in conjunction with the clinical forensic medicine section of the Royal Society of Medicine. With all these training facilities available, the novice police surgeon should be able to obtain the DMJ in between three and five years. This postgraduate qualification is one of the few means by which those actively engaged in medicolegal work may expect instant recognition as experts in this speciality of medical practice. Details summarising various training facilities and forensic societies are given at the end of the chapter.

A calendar of one-day courses held at other centres throughout the UK and details of overseas forensic meetings are published in the APS News, sent twice a year to APS members. Finally, police surgeons often work in isolation and it behoves any doctor on becoming appointed to join the APS.

The Association of Police Surgeons

Most police surgeons belong to the APS (address given at the end of the chapter), whose membership offers the following benefits.

- The APS is solely concerned with the furtherance of clinical forensic medicine in general and the interests of members in particular.

- The APS, in conjunction with the BMA, negotiates the best possible terms of service.

- Members are kept informed of APS-recommended meetings, essential for acquiring basic knowledge, keeping up to date and providing opportunities for informal contact with national and international authorities.

- Members receive free copies of the APS Diary and Journals (*The Journal of Clinical Forensic Medicine*, published four times a year, and the *APS News* published twice a year).

- The APS publishes textbooks and monographs. Well-illustrated monographs on *Rape* and *Non-accidental injury in children* are currently available.

- The APS supplies inexpensive examination aids, for example clinical record proformas and anatomical charts.

- The APS subscription is tax allowable.

- Full membership gives voting rights on policy matters and Council representation.

- The APS enjoys a close working relationship with representatives of allied disciplines at home and abroad, for example police officers, forensic scientists, forensic pathologists and lawyers.

- As the most influential voice of police surgeons in the UK, the APS is frequently consulted on matters relating to clinical forensic medicine.

- The APS is non-political and non-sectarian.

Training opportunities

Initial training

National Training Centre for Scientific Support to Crime Investigation, Durham Constabulary

Enquiries to: Dr N. Weston, Harperley Hall, Crook, County Durham DL15 8DS

Tel: 01388–762191

The Metropolitan Police have their own training courses at the Police Training Centre, Hendon, Middlesex.

Enquiries to: Dr F Lewington, Metropolitan Police Forensic Science Laboratory, 109 Lambeth Road, London   SE1 7PL

Tel: 0171–230 6308

Development training

Forensic Academy Group in the North (FAGIN)

Enquiries to: Dr S Robinson, Rose

Cottage, Sunbank Lane, Ringway, Cheshire   WA15 0PZ

Tel: 0161–980 1498

South East and London Group (SEAL)

Enquiries to: Dr F Lewington (see above)

Meetings are held monthly at the Metropolitan Police Forensic Science Laboratory.

Avon and Somerset Constabulary

Enquiries to: Dr R Bunting, Force Medical Officer, Occupational Health Unit, Avon & Somerset Constabulary, Napier Miles House, Napier Miles Road, Kings Weston, Bristol   BS11 0UT

Tel: 01272–454358

Meetings are held usually at weekends (three or four per year) in West Country hotels.

Useful addresses

Association of Police Surgeons
18A Mount Parade,
Harrogate
North Yorkshire   HG1 1BX

Tel: 01423–509727
Fax: 01423–566391

Dr WDS McLay OBE
Chief Medical Officer
Strathclyde Police
173 Pitt Street
Glasgow G2 4JS

Tel: 0141–204 2626

BMA Forensic Medicine Sub-committee
BMA House
Tavistock Square
London   WC1 9JP

Tel: 0171–387 4499
Fax: 0171–383 6406

Metropolitan Police
Manager, FME Service
SO 20 Branch, Room 1509
New Scotland Yard
Broadway
London   SW1H 0BG

Tel: 0171–230 3854

7　The role of the part-time prison medical officer

Eric Godfrey

The Prison Service serves the public by keeping in custody those committed by the courts. It is society's duty is to look after them with humanity and help them to lead law-abiding and useful lives, both in custody and after release.

The Prison Service in England and Wales is responsible for some 50 000 individuals detained or remanded in approximately 130 prison establishments. Prison inmates may be transferred between establishments, depending on custodial reasons, such as length of sentence and the degree of security considered suitable. Young inmates are detained in Young Offenders Institutions.

The aim of the Prison Service's Health Care Directorate is that the health care needs of prisoners should be met at a standard at least equal to that of the NHS. It is vital, therefore, for the Prison Service to attract and maintain a sufficient number of high-calibre GPs to provide part-time medical services, to ensure that the primary care element of this aim is met.

Each prisoner undergoes an assessment of physical and mental health by a doctor within 24 hours of arrival at a prison. This assessment ensures that those needing management of physical or mental illness, or drug rehabilitation, are suitably identified. New entrants to prison undergo an assessment of physical and mental health before a medical recommendation is made about where they should be located within the prison. Prison staff are trained to be alert to the tell-tale signs of depression as part of a suicide awareness programme.

Where appropriate, referral to NHS facilities can be arranged. For some, medical and psychiatric reports are required for court.

Prison Medical Officers (PMOs) provide morning surgeries but may also undertake longer assessments of complex problems. In addition, PMOs have statutory duties of visiting segregated prisoners and of assessing the physical and mental state of prisoners facing disciplinary charges, in a process known as adjudication.

The management and surveillance of chronic disease as a positive approach to health promotion is undertaken by doctors and health care staff. The health care centre in prisons are staffed by prison officers specialising in health care, as well as by general nurses trained in psychiatric nursing. Health care centres include the provision of pharmacy, optical and dental services.

Minor surgery may be offered in the prison health care centre, or arrangements may be made for attendance at an NHS hospital. Immunisation programmes, particularly for hepatitis B are offered. All inmates are offered education on HIV/AIDS. Many establishments have visiting consultants in genitourinary medicine. A substantial proportion of inmates have abused drugs, and detoxification is undertaken either within the health care centre or on location in the prison.

Prison establishments have a number of distinct roles. All male adult prisoners (over 21 years of age) first enter 'local' prisons near their own homes. Women's prisons are fewer in number, and because of this, some women prisoners cannot be accommodated near their homes. Longer-term prisoners may be transferred to training prisons, where longer sentences are served. Open prisons are establishments where non-violent prisoners and those near the end of their sentences may be kept in custody prior to their final release. Remand centres house those prisoners who have not been convicted. Offenders under the age of 21 are located in young offenders institutions.

Working as a part-time PMO is far from routine. One will face and manage a wide range of activities and situations, many of which may not have been encountered before. A series of induction courses and seminars, which are supported by a growing commitment to continuing medical education, should help to ensure the necessary knowledge and skills to perform this challenging and demanding work.

Practitioners outside the Prison Service often assume that the age span of prisoners means that there is little in the way of 'illness'. On the contrary, as well as the problems that are met in general practice, there is much to be uncovered in the way of chronic illness, both mental and physical.

Many prisoners have led disorganised and chaotic lives, with alcohol and drugs playing a major role, and have suffered the consequences of the neglect of their health.

One area of the GP's knowledge that will be expanded is psychiatry, not only in diagnosing psychopathy, but also in recognising when a psychopathy flips into a psychotic state. Expressions of depression are common, but true depressive states have to be differentiated from despondency and 'fed-upness' in many prisoners. One will occasionally recognise a temporal lobe epileptic state that may not have been previously diagnosed, and, where appropriate, treatment can totally alter behaviour.

Physical conditions are also common. For example, neglect, chronic chest infection, hypertension and heart disease, anaemia, diabetes and genito-urinary infections will all be found. One of the great attractions of working in a prison is that the health care team will also include registered nurses or hospital officers (disciplined staff who have undergone nursing training), who will assist in providing care to inmates in the health care centre. Many prisons now have inpatient bed facilities in the health care centre, which allows the GP to monitor a patient's condition.

The work of a PMO can be clearly divided into three categories. First, the provision of normal clinical care, as in NHS practice. Second, work that relates directly to the forensic or legal aspects of practice, which includes the assessment of the prisoners' physical and mental health before 'adjudication', the means by which the Governor administers punishment for offences against prison rules. Third, work that can be broadly described as management, in which the PMO advises the Governor or manages the provision of health care, including budgetary advice or management and the employment of visiting consultants and other health professionals. Where mental illness requires hospital treatment, transfer, generally under the Mental Health Act, to an NHS hospital may be undertaken. Prisoners who have arrived at the prison during the day normally undergo their reception medical examination on the evening of the day of their arrival.

Surgeries or sick parades are scheduled for a time agreed by the doctor and the Governor, on behalf of prison officers. Part-time PMOs, will be expected to respond to emergencies as in their own NHS practice. In addition, arrangements need to be made for on-call cover on a rota basis. Depending on the size and function of the prison, health care centres are staffed either for 24 hours a day or for a shorter time, so that hours of attendance are determined locally.

GPs acting as part-time PMOs have normally been expected to make arrangements with partners for on-call cover and remuneration agreed for a notional number of hours to reflect the work-load. In addition, a flat rate on-call allowance and a call-out fee are payable. This is, at the present time, an area subject to negotiation between the BMA and the Prison Service.

Being able to work as part of a team is crucial to the role of part-time PMOs; this makes NHS GPs ideal individuals, given the nature of their work within partnerships. Apart from physicians, dentists, opticians and chiropodists, there will be the support team of psychiatrists, psychologists, the Probation Service, staff, the After-Care Service, duty specialists, educationalists and others, all of whom will have the aim of preparing the prisoner for a better life when released.

Apart from general medical services, there are specific areas in which the

GP's skills will be needed, for example the necessity for segregation, fitness for work, disciplinary action, recognition that prisoners may be under the influence of drugs, parole reports, reports to court and answering questions from relatives, Members of Parliament and prison visitors. This may sound substantial but, thankfully, these demands do not all come at once.

Under the existing arrangements, a part-time PMO's contract places an obligation on the doctor to provide cover during annual leave; most doctors are able to ask their partners to provide cover. This particular arrangement is currently subject to negotiation between the BMA and the Prison Service, with the aim of transferring the responsibility for finding and providing locum cover from the part-time PMO to the prison Governor.

Until recently, a part-time PMO could only gain advancement by undertaking the role of Managing Medical Officer. However, negotiations are already underway that would make it possible for a doctor to become better paid by demonstrating the acquisition of specialist skills achieved via gaining the proposed Three Royal Colleges Diploma in Prison Medicine. The Prison Service is aware of the need to recognise and reward the clinical skills and experience of these doctors. An incremental salary scale based on length of service was introduced during 1995.

There are currently some 125 doctors contracted to provide part-time medical services. Bearing in mind that many share their duties with partners or locums, perhaps as many as 300 GPs provide some input into the care of patients in prisons. The number of hours contracted by part-time medical officers varies from 7 to 30 hours per week, with an average of about 12 hours.

The responsibility of a part-time PMO to the patient is no different from that which would apply outside the prison. The role of the doctor is never punitive or custodial. Restraint is only ever justifiable as part of the treatment of illness, and consent for treatment is the same as in circumstances outside prison. The compulsory treatment of mental illness is allowed in a hospital only under the Mental Health Act. For the purposes of the Act, a prison health care centre is not a hospital. If a prisoner is judged to be in need of hospital treatment, it must be provided in a hospital. This may be in a regional secure unit or in one of the hospitals of the Special Hospital Authority (Broadmoor, Ashworth or Rampton).

The prison Governor has overall responsibility for the provision of health care in the prison. Good working relationships contribute greatly to the effectiveness of delivery, and health care is only one of the Governor's wide areas of responsibility. Good health care delivered within budget does much to enhance the reputation of the prison and the service, as well as meeting the stated aims and objectives of the Prison Service. Part-time PMOs are responsible for pointing out to the Governor factors affecting the health of both prisoners and staff working within the prison. These factors will vary between prisons. In any organisation subject to change, a conscientious doctor will recognise the importance of health care in the totality of the role of the prison, and will expect to attend and contribute advice and expertise to the Governor on a regular basis, taking pride in the quality of such aspects of medical practice. The adage 'manage or be managed' applies equally within prisons. Doctors are now familiar with business plans, strategic planning and budgeting in a way that would have been unusual in clinical specialties only a few years ago.

The Prison Service has committed itself to recognising the special nature of medical work in prisons. This explains its support for the proposals from the medical Royal Colleges that the specialty become recognised through the creation of a Diploma in Prison Medicine, for which teaching modules have already begun. It is hoped that the first diplomas will be granted in 1997. Doctors in the Prison Service will eventually be offered up to 60 days instruction and training during the first three years in the Service. Attainment of the diploma will be regarded as a career advancement, which would attract a higher salary and increased prospects of promotion.

Work in the Prison Service on a part-time basis is not superannuable either under the civil service pension scheme or the NHS. Doctors may therefore wish to seek specialist advice concerning the purchase of a private pension for this portion of their income.

It is important that all partners involved in the provision of services to a prison share a commitment to provide quality medical care to those who have been detained. The NHS (General Medical Services) Regulations 1992 place an obligation on GPs to provide a minimum commitment to satisfy the requirements of their FHSA. GPs working as part-time PMOs should ensure that their position is not compromised in delivering their NHS commitments. It is also important that the prison is prepared to be flexible and to understand the obligations of a part-time PMO to meet responsibilities outside the prison, as well as inside. It is therefore difficult for a single-handed doctor to join the Prison Service, especially in view of the 1990 contract. For doctors in partnership, there must be the willing co-operation of practice colleagues to be prepared to share some of the work-load.

Having read all the above, you may wonder why you should even consider joining the Service. Apart from any altruistic motives, proposals for new contracts for Prison Medical Officers, both full time and part time are under discussion. The pay and terms of service are currently (1995) being negotiated, and will be a great improvement from what is presently available; they may also for the first time, be pensionable.

The Prison Service review of medical staffing and remuneration for both full- and part-time PMOs is underway. The BMA will be closely involved in these discussions to ensure that the interests of part-time PMOs are firmly protected. These changes are not expected to come into effect until at least early 1997. GPs who are interested in joining the Prison Service should, however, in the meantime contact their **local** BMA office for up-to-date guidance.

8 Working for schools and colleges

Roger Harrington

The way in which health care is provided for pupils in schools depends largely on whether the school in question is maintained or independent, day or boarding. There are considerable differences between the varying institutions, and, ideally, every school should have a nominated medical officer. In practice, the vast majority of maintained schools are day-only, with the pupils receiving their medical care from the school health service, while most boarding schools are found in the independent sector.

Historical perspectives

The belief that universal education would result in a general improvement in people's health was a fundamental part of the philosophy of the Victorian pioneers of the public health service in Great Britain. In 1870, only half the children of school age were in school, and from then onwards, it became increasingly evident that a general improvement in health was necessary before the majority of children could take advantage of the educational services offered. Many children were disabled by ill health and poor feeding, to the extent that they were unable to benefit from school, and, indeed, the average young recruit to the Boer War was noted to be in poor physical shape. Legislation affecting the health of school children was introduced in 1906 when Local Education Authorities (LEAs) were empowered to provide meals. The following year, the Education Act enabled LEAs to provide for the medical inspection of school children and to make provision for attending to their health and physical condition. The first school clinic opened in Bradford in 1908, and, in the early years, the service was concerned with the treatment of defects found at school medical inspections that could not be treated adequately elsewhere.

The Education Act of 1918 laid a duty on LEAs to provide for the medical inspection and treatment of illness in children in elementary schools, and empowered them to arrange for the treatment of children in secondary schools. RA Butler's famous 1944 Act required LEAs to provide school meals and milk for pupils at schools they maintained, medical and dental inspections in all types of maintained schools and all forms of medical and dental treatment, without cost to the parents. With the inception of the NHS in 1948, recognition was made of the community health services provided by local authorities for children in schools and for those under five years of age, but these services remained under the control of local government.

With the reorganisation of the NHS in 1974, responsibility for the school health service was transferred from LEAs to the then Area Health Authorities (AHAs) who were required to provide facilities for the medical examination of children in schools, especially those needing special examination and treatment. The subsequent restructuring of the NHS in 1982, when the AHAs were abolished, gave responsibility for the service to health authorities (HAs).

Provision of medical care

HAs now manage all the community health services for the population in their areas and employ clinical medical officers (CMOs), who may visit a number of schools carrying out varying tasks, such as routine medical examinations and the administration of vaccinations. In such schools, CMOs do not prescribe treatment but should maintain close contact with the pupils' own family doctors, either directly or via the consultant community paediatrician.

In contrast, doctors appointed to independent schools are usually GPs who are contracted to the local FHSA for the provision of general medical services to those patients on their NHS list. By implication, pupils attending a day school will be from the surrounding area, and it is more likely that they will have their own GPs. In such situations, they would not be registered with the school doctor, although he or she would have responsibility for them during their time at school. The opposite situation arises in boarding schools, where pupils may be from different parts of the UK or from abroad. Although it is convenient for all pupils to be registered with the nominated school medical officer, the 1989 Children Act states that all pupils should have the opportunity to register with a GP of their own choice, particularly one of the same gender.

Academic, administrative and domestic staff (and their dependants), as well as the pupils, may register with the school doctor, who is therefore responsible for providing medical services during both term and school holidays if this group of patients is resident in the school area. NHS guidelines, issued in 1994, confirm that it is the school, rather than the parental address that determines the residence of the pupil with regard to the purchasing of hospital services by either the relevant HA or the school doctor as a fundholding GP.

The school doctor's work

While this work is varied, it is, essentially, an extension of a GP's practice work, with similar duties, responsibilities and problems. In contrast to general medical services, the school doctor deals with children of a specific age range, for example 5 – 13 years or 13 – 18 years, who are generally healthy individuals. The work may be divided into acute and routine; in the former group, there is a high prevalence of respiratory tract infections and sporting injuries. In the latter group, the school doctor may be concerned with activities such as carrying out periodical medical examinations and maintaining vaccination programmes.

In addition to NHS contractual obligations, an independent school doctor is responsible for a range of other duties including:

- advising head teachers and governing bodies on matters concerning the health of staff and pupils

- discussing the health and fitness of individual pupils with house masters, house mistresses and other staff, subject to the constraints of confidentiality

- supervising the sanatorium or sick bay, and advising on the appointment of nursing staff and their professional duties

- periodically examining pupils, including screening for visual and hearing defects and monitoring physical development

- establishing epidemiological surveillance

- arranging immunisation programmes and ensuring that all pupils are immunised in accordance with current practice, as recommended by the DoH

- maintaining communication with parents with regard to medical investigations, treatment and immunisations of pupils, subject to the constraints of confidentiality

- collaborating with the head teacher and governing body and, when applicable, the Environmental Health Officer regarding the hygiene of the school premises

- giving advice on the prevention of accidents and sporting injuries, including requirements under the Health and Safety at Work (etc) Act

- advising the school and the delegated member of staff on matters relating to the regulations concerned with the Control of Substances Hazardous to Health (COSHH) regulations

- ensuring that pupils receive regular dental inspections and any necessary treatment, either at school or through their parents or guardians

- arranging for the pre-employment medical examinations of teaching and non-teaching staff, and advising the head teacher and governing body accordingly

- providing certificates of incapacity to work, as required by the school, in respect of its employees

- providing international certificates of vaccination where necessary

- providing certificates for fitness or freedom from infection for participation in school trips, travel and employment

- provision of reports for university medical officers and certificates of fitness to attend university or colleges of further education

- completion of claim forms for private health insurance benefit.

These are wide-ranging and comprehensive services, which school doctors should aim to provide to the fullest. It is vital that there is a contract between the school and the doctor, outlining the conditions of his or her employment and covering such issues as expected duties, remuneration, required notice in the event of resignation, retirement age and grievance procedures.

Medical services in schools

In day schools, it is essential that at least a sick room is provided where pupils who are taken ill or injured at school can rest and be treated before they go home. The room should be quiet and warm and should, as a minimum contain a bed, table, chair, washbasin and lavatory facilities. A locked cupboard should be provided, which is accessible to the school nurse or a responsible member of staff, containing a basic first aid kit and simple remedies such as paracetamol. In consultation with the school medical officer, protocols should be drawn up to allow the nurse or staff member to administer medication to pupils requiring it, and a policy should be in place regarding the administration of prescribed medicines, for example courses of antibiotics, to pupils while in school.

Boarding schools should have their own sanatorium or sick bay, staffed by trained personnel, thereby allowing the schools medical and nursing services to be in one location. The nurse in charge of a sanatorium should be either a registered general nurse (RGN) or a registered sick children's nurse (RSCN). Twenty-four hour cover of the sanatorium, is desirable but some institutions may, because of financial constraints, operate a policy of being open during 'office hours', with an 'on-call' system at other times. The staffing levels should be such that there is adequate off-duty cover, particularly if a 24-hour service is offered.

The design of the school medical room will inevitably reflect the accommodation available and the requirements of a particular school. The number of beds available will vary from school to school, depending on the number of boarders, the age range of the pupils, whether or not the school is single sex or co-educational, the availability of sick room facilities within houses, and the proximity of local district general hospitals. Most boarding schools have a wide variety of outdoor and sporting activities, and there should be a room adjacent to the school doctor's consulting room that is available for acute injuries and for injured pupils awaiting transport to either hospital or their home.

Nursing staff who are resident in the school should have adequate accommodation to reflect the fact that the school is their home. Additionally, staff who share an on-call rota should have sleeping, washing and lavatory facilities provided.

Commitment

The time commitment for a school doctor will vary, depending on the school size, the requirements of the head teacher and governing body, and the doctor's own enthusiasm and level of expertise. It may be convenient to hold a regular surgery at the school, the frequency of which may range from daily for up to two hours, to three times weekly or even once weekly. The school doctor should be mindful of the academic timetable and ensure that his or her surgeries are held outside lesson times or, if this is not feasible, timed to cause minimal disruption. Similarly, by liaising with the appointment staff at his or her local hospital, the school doctor can try to ensure that outpatient appointments are arranged for the most convenient times. Wherever possible, routine matters such as dental check-ups should be arranged during the school holidays.

There will obviously be an 'on-call' commitment that a school doctor, in partnership with other GPs, will share with his colleagues. School doctors contemplating joining co-operatives or deputising services should be aware of their contractual obligations to the school and ensure that any new on-call arrangements are agreeable to the head teacher and governing body. While it can be argued that a refreshed school doctor who has not had a disturbed night on duty will be of more value to the school, it must be recognised that many schools feel that, as they are paying for the services of a particular doctor, a total stranger with no knowledge of the environment or the pupils is unacceptable.

Some of the school doctor's work is 'seasonal', the winter term providing a heavy work-load of sporting injuries from the rugby and soccer fields. With the possibility of a number of school teams playing different sports at home, a winter Saturday can be particularly onerous for the school doctor or his on-call colleague. The spring term is often characterized by outbreaks of viral respiratory tract infections, while the summer months provide seasonal allergies such as hayfever and problems relating to impending public examinations. New entrant medical examinations and the routine updating of vaccinations may require the arranging of extra sessions, while an annual health and hygiene inspection of the school premises, frequent meetings with the headteacher, involvement in the school's health education programme and, perhaps, the provision of first aid lectures to staff and pupils all make extra demands on the school doctor's time.

Remuneration

The school doctor employed by a HA and working in the maintained sector would be remunerated in accordance with national pay scales, although the prospect of local pay bargaining is looming, and school doctors will presumably not be immune from this. The doctor in the independent sector is paid by the school authorities and may be remunerated in one of two ways. For schools with a large number of pupils, for example greater than 300, the doctor may be paid on a sessional basis in accordance with rates of pay for part-time occupational health physicians. Such rates are available from **local**

BMA offices and are revised annually in accordance with the recommendations of the DDRB.

For smaller institutions, the doctor may be paid a so-called 'suggested fee', published annually by the BMA. This is a sum paid annually per boarding pupil and is in addition to any fees and allowances that the doctor earns by virtue of his or her NHS work for the school. The BMA suggested fee for 1995/96 is £31 per pupil per annum. This is not a binding fee but merely a guideline to assist doctors and their schools in their pay negotiations. Ideally, every school doctor should be paid the full suggested fee, but in practice few are. When negotiating with the school, the doctor should take into account not only the amount of work involved, but also other factors, such as the kudos of being the school doctor, the free use of such sporting facilities as squash courts, swimming pools and golf courses, and any fee discounts should the doctor wish to educate his or her own children at the particular establishment. Some school doctors in partnership consider that it is unfair that they alone should attract the financial advantage of a fee discount and either strive for their colleagues to receive similar advantages or try to opt for a higher 'suggested fee' and a lower discount, with the aim of pooling the money and thus benefiting all their colleagues.

Training

While there is no formal training for school doctors, experience in paediatrics, accident and emergency medicine, psychiatry and general practice is clearly desirable. Although there is no substitute for an experienced GP who has developed the necessary communication skills, those holding the MRCGP, DCH or DCCH might have achieved higher academic standards.

For any doctor who is comfortable dealing with young people and their particular problems, schools medicine can be rich and rewarding. Although the time commitment may be high, the non-financial rewards can be considerable. However, nationally, there has been a 20% decline in boarding places, in the last ten years, which has diminished opportunities for doctors to become school medical officers.

There is a great deal of job satisfaction, and the school doctor can become an integral part of the school community. It is possible to become involved in much of the day-to-day life of the school, such as concerts, staff plays and sporting activities, and it can be immensely satisfying to follow a pupil's progress from entry to leaving, either going on to a senior school at the age of 13 or on to employment or further education at 18 or 19 years of age.

Medical Officers of Schools Association

MOSA was founded in 1884 with the original objects of 'assisting members in promoting school hygiene' and 'holding meetings for the consideration of all subjects connected with the special work of medical officers of schools'. Nowadays, it represents doctors working in either the maintained or independent education sector but having, as a common goal, the health of the school child. Currently, there are approximately 450 members, and it is administered by a Council consisting of Officers, Past Presidents and up to 24 other members of the Association. Twice-yearly meetings are held for members, in the form of an all-day or weekend residential meeting in January and a summer meeting at a school. Both gatherings include academic topics relevant to schools medicine, and members receive a quarterly newsletter outlining current trends. The Honorary Secretary also runs an advisory service to help both members and non-members with any aspect of their school work, including clinical, financial, contractual and ethical matters.

Further reading

Faculty of Community Health of the Society of Public Health Limited. *The School Health Service.*

Medical Officers of Schools Association (1992) *Handbook of School Health*, 17th edn. Trentham Books.

Useful address

Medical Officers of Schools Association
c/o The Medical Society of London
11 Chandos Street
London W1

9 Pharmaceutical trials

Frank Wells

New medicines cannot be made available until a great deal of research that satisfies the licensing authority has been carried out. In the UK, the licensing authority is the Medicines Control Agency (acting on behalf of the Secretary of State for Health). Since 1 January 1995 there has also been a European licensing authority, known as the European Medicines Evaluation Agency (acting on behalf of the European Commission).

As well as the research needed before a product licence can be granted, further research may also be required after such a licence has been issued. Every medicine is licensed on the grounds of safety, efficacy and quality, but much more experience may be needed on the way in which the licensed medicine behaves in clinical practice than is available at the licensing stage. Thus, further research may be needed to establish a realistic safety database for the medicine in question.

Expenditure on research and development

The total amount of money that the pharmaceutical industry in the UK spends on research and development is impressive: on average, for each of the last three years (1992–94) for which figures are available, expenditure was in the region of £1.5 billion. The total UK pharmaceutical industry includes the UK subsidiaries of multinational overseas companies, as well as the UK parent companies themselves, which include Glaxo/Wellcome, SmithKline Beecham and Zeneca.

Threats to research

It is a significant achievement that five of the top 15 medicines currently in use worldwide were discovered in the UK; much of the clinical evaluation of the remaining medicines was also undertaken in the UK. However, certain trends indicate that the position of the UK as a country in which the international pharmaceutical industry is confident to invest and place clinical research projects may be under threat. These threats include the effects of both the general economic climate affecting the UK and the emphasis on the costs of medicines (in the NHS). This emphasis is understandably having a measurable effect on the prescribing of branded products marketed by those very companies that are actually conducting or sponsoring research. From a multinational industry point of view, this is beginning to undermine confidence in what is happening in the UK.

Fields of clinical research

Despite these threats, the list of fields in which research of any kind is being conducted in the UK remains impressive. The current avenues of research and development in the acute field include AIDS, new treatments for cancer, more effective treatments for cardiovascular and respiratory disease, treatments to arrest the complications of diabetes and extensive research into biotechnology. Additionally, British research is currently being conducted into treatment for different types of anaemia, Alzheimer's disease, anxiety disorders and depression, leprosy, worm infestations and other diseases of developing countries, Huntington's chorea, Parkinson's disease, anorexia and schizophrenia, some of them of minimal direct interest to general practice but demonstrating that pharmaceutical companies also have an interest in Third World problems. We can be reasonably satisfied of the achievements already made, and particularly of the commitments given to furthering advances in treatment.

Factors influencing research investment

Other factors impinge on the conduct of clinical research that are of direct relevance to general practice. The first of these is the definitive version of the European Good Clinical Research Practice (GCP – not GCRP) guidelines, which requires that certain standards are met, of which investigators must be aware so that they know what is expected of them. For many years, the UK pharmaceutical industry has had similar voluntary standards, but as these guidelines have now become requirements, anyone involved in clinical research throughout Europe must be aware of them.

Good Clinical Research Practice

The important principles of GCRP set standards to which the research-based pharmaceutical industry is wholly committed. In 1988, the Association of British Pharmaceutical Industries (ABPI) issued its definitive policy on Good Clinical Research Practice, which has proved invaluable during discussions and negotiations building up to the publication of a European Commission directive on the same subject (91/507/EEC). Guidelines on clinical research apply to all four phases of clinical research:

- Phase I – Clinical pharmacology studies, using non-patient volunteers. They follow on after laboratory and animal or toxicological studies, the results of which must be satisfactory before a new substance is first given to human beings.

- Phase II – Pilot studies in which potential medicines are first given to patients.

- Phase III – Full-scale clinical trials, conducted on patients, to establish the efficacy and, to a limited extent, the safety of a new medicine. The results of Phase III studies, if successful, will be used in the dossier submitted with a product licence application to the licensing authority.

- Phase IV – Studies conducted after a licence has been granted and the product has been marketed.

Additionally, observational studies may be undertaken to assess the safety of marketed medicines, but these should not be confused with clinical trials that involve a degree of intervention, as far as patients are concerned, over and above normal prescribing practice. Anything extra that is described in the protocol – such as the completion of diary cards, or the requirement for extra blood tests or ECGs, for example – means that the study is a Phase IV clinical trial, with all that this involves regarding ethical approval and informed consent, rather than an observational cohort study. Such studies are covered by the Safety Assessment of Marketed Medicines (SAMM) guidelines, produced by the ABPI in collaboration with the BMA, the Committee on Safety of Medicines (CSM) the Medicines Control Agency (MCA) and the Royal College of General Practitioners (RCGP).

GCP guidelines

Since the introduction of the EC directive referred to above, clear guidelines on the principles of GCP have been adopted for all clinical trials sponsored by pharmaceutical companies. A card setting out the responsibilities of investigators conducting trials to GCP standards is available from the ABPI, as are separate cards setting out guidelines for Phase IV clinical trials, investigator site audits and clinical trial compensation.

Certain items are emphasized in the GCP guidelines. First, they cover the selection of investigators and of centres where a research project is going to be conducted. The criteria to be considered include the experience of the investigator; the location of any centre, be it hospital, contract research organisation or general practice; the facilities and staff available; the commitment or otherwise of the investigator actually to conduct the study within his or her normal clinical commitment; the existence of an adequate subject population from which the study subjects may be drawn; and the special need, if the study is to be a multicentre one, to identify a co-ordinator either from within the company or amongst the investigators. Of great importance is the role of the local research ethics committee, to which further attention is given below.

Second, the protocol for a proposed study must be discussed with a potential investigator. The detailed protocol should follow rather than precede initial discussions with potential investigators, and in any event should meet a number of requirements. While this is crucial, it is often short-circuited. The ABPI guidelines set out a checklist of the items to be included in a protocol, but particular emphasis is given to the need for effective monitoring, and auditing, of a trial, which will require access to original source documents. This does not mean snooping round the hospital or GP surgery, looking into the complete histories in patient's notes; it means doing whatever is necessary to satisfy the monitor or auditor that what is written in the clinical report forms is true. This can invariably be achieved in ways that preserve adequate patient confidentiality.

Apart from the protocol, it is essential to have a formal agreement between the sponsoring company, or the contract house conducting the trial on behalf of a company, and the investigator. It is only right and proper that a doctor who has agreed to fulfil a protocol – and similarly a company or contract house that has agreed to fulfil its responsibilities as set out in a protocol – should feel that this commitment is absolute, and that appropriate sanctions should apply if the protocol is violated during the conduct of the study. The obvious first sanction to be taken against an investigator who underachieves is not to pay the full amount of money to which he or she would otherwise be entitled. No-one gains if that happens although no-one really loses either, but that is not an adequate sanction when it comes to misconduct or even fraud. Then it is necessary to take further action; fortunately, this situation is now rarely met.

Ethics committees

The ethical approval of a clinical trial protocol is essential and must always be obtained before any clinical trial is begun. The ethical approval of the investigator is also important, and the industry is committed to ensuring that this happens. Obviously, if a trial is being conducted in a single centre, the local research ethics committee (LREC) is able to consider the protocol and the investigator at the same time, but in a multicentre trial, where it may be acceptable to obtain ethical approval from a single committee, such as that operated by the RCGP under the chairmanship of Sir Michael Drury, the investigator's LREC must also be involved, exercising its duty to ensure that it agrees with the ethical approval of the protocol, and taking prime responsibility for approving the investigator. The effectiveness of LRECs across the country, however, has been very variable, although steps are currently being taken by the DoH and others to improve the position.

Consent

The purpose of informed consent is to make sure that anyone who is the subject of a clinical trial is fully aware of what the clinical trial involves, and of his or her own rights and responsibilities within that clinical trial. No pharmaceutical company worth its salt is going to encourage anything less than this. It should be written, or at the very least witnessed if not written. The elements of informed consent are important, and include being given information about all known and foreseeable risks and discomforts, as well as about all known benefits, which, of course, in the context of a clinical trial may well be none at all. The data arising from a trial must be confidential, although the subject must know that the data and record forms might have to be disclosed to a regulatory authority; this has caused little difficulty, in practice. As already mentioned, there must be proper compensation arrangements in place for medicine-induced injury in the course of a clinical trial. It is important to remind patients that their participation really is voluntary and that they may withdraw at any time without prejudice to their continued medical care. One of the more contentious elements of informed consent on which there is an ABPI policy is the need to have a 24-hour contact telephone number so that any queries arising can be answered immediately.

Monitoring of clinical studies

The whole question of the monitoring of clinical trials is a pivotal part of the European guidelines on GCP, and it features prominently in the ABPI guidelines. The overall progress of a study, including the rate of recruitment and the completeness of the clinical record forms, has to be constantly assessed. Sometimes, standards are seen to have slipped; doctors must be aware of the absolute need to maintain high standards when they take part as clinical trial investigators, their training in the principles of GCP is essential.

Remuneration

Payment for participation in clinical trials sponsored by pharmaceutical companies is usually based on the fees guidance published by the BMA. The current (1995) suggested pro rata fee is £116.50 per hour. Companies are well able to assess accurately how long investigator assessments will take and can budget accordingly. They will take into account such matters as overheads, laboratory and other expenses, the involvement of secondary investigators, such as ECG technicians and practice nurses, and the involvement of pharmacists. These considerations are, of course, over and above the basic fee to which the investigator is entitled. Typically, therefore, a fully trained GP investigator may be asked to take part in a clinical trial in which he is expected to see each patient-subject six times for 20 minutes each time, after an initial 30-minute recruitment assessment. He may be asked to recruit six patients, within eight weeks, and to have completed the study within six months. If he succeeds in recruiting five patients within the allotted time, and completes their assessments within six months, he is thus entitled to (using the BMA's [1995] suggested fee of £116.50 per hour) £116.50 × 2.5 × 5

= £1456.25. An experienced investigator might undertake ten studies in a year, and thus earn in the region of £15 000.

Other fees to which a doctor is entitled in the clinical research context are a fee for confirming that a non-patient volunteer has no medical reason, known to the GP, for not taking part in a Phase I study (which is an extract from the medical records), and those for involvement in SAMM studies, which vary depending on the complexity of the form to be completed.

Conclusions

GPs, the community and pharmaceutical companies can mutually benefit from clinical research, and it is essential in the development of effective new medicines. The work involved is arduous, because of the safeguards that exist, which were largely put in place voluntarily by the pharmaceutical industry, regarding research projects. However, it can also be exciting and intellectually, as well as financially, rewarding. GPs interested in pursuing this field of activity should contact the medical directors of major pharmaceutical companies with a known involvement in the therapeutic categories of particular interest to the doctor. Further information, and the guidelines issued by the ABPI referred to in this chapter, can be obtained from the author.

10   Part-time occupational health work

Joe Kearns

The Health of the Nation noted 'The increasing concern of employers and their workforces to improve health offers opportunities to develop and increase such activity in the workplace.'[1] Priority targets were set for preventive medicine. Ten options for action were offered to management. While they are generally concerned with the promotion of health, three of them concern health, safety and welfare. Health promotion activity in the work-place is concerned with using opportunities in that setting to promote healthy life-styles, behaviour and attitudes in everyday life outside work. Within that preventive scope, occupational health is a distinct discipline, covering the effects of work conditions on people's health and of employees' health status on their own and others' health and safety at work.

Box 10.1: Occupational health is involved in:

- setting up management systems to recognise risks

- identifying and controlling known hazards to health

- providing first aid

- helping in the rehabilitation of employees after illness or injury

- developing policies to identify and deal with employees' problems

- providing information, instruction and training to employers and employees on health and safety.

Recent, more detailed guidance on occupational health services in the NHS suggests that one that 'has demonstrable competence can provide the basis for a service to other employers'. Adopting that principle, a general practice would be well advised to be confident of its own competence in the field before offering specialist advice to others.

In the past, medical or nursing care at the place of work was often regarded as a welfare provision for the benefit of staff. Managers in small enterprises have a vague sense of a need for medical help and frequently invite a doctor to visit their premises from time to time. Particularly in smaller communities, the visiting doctor might be expected to provide general medical care to employees on a factory site, perhaps with the aid of a nurse. That is no longer a satisfactory arrangement for either party. Legislation now requires the employer to assess all the activities undertaken by employees, on or off site, for risk. If medical arrangements have to be made to deal adequately and competently with those risks, occupational health skills must be added to the usual general medical or nursing competence of the doctor or the nurse. It is important to have a clear job description and contract specifying the expertise and information required and offered by each side, since the doctor may otherwise unwittingly be assumed to have not only clinical responsibility, but also liability in relation to risks that the employer has failed to identify. The duty of the occupational physician is primarily to protect the health of the worker, while also acting as a medical resource to management.

Box 10.2: Management of health and safety

In 1992, the booklet *Successful management of health and safety* published by the Health and Safety Executive (HSE), emphasised that health and safety issues are to be integrated into the competent management of any enterprise employing five or more people in the public or private sector. Most general practices are within the scope of the associated legislation. The NHS Executive document on health and safety [HSG(94)51] provides a wider review of the scope of statutory imperatives previously obscured by Crown Immunity.

The legal context

A fundamental principle of the Health and Safety at Work (etc) Act 1974 is the expectation that the employer (including the NHS authority, Trust or individual general practice) must, as far as is reasonably practicable, make the work-place safe for employees, contractors and members of the public. The Act began a process by which earlier prescriptive regulation of limited sectors of industry, such as the Factories Act (1961) or the Offices, Shops and Railway Premises Act (1963), affecting 'occupiers', gave way to the requirement that all employers should implement general principles intended to protect the health and safety of all their employees, contractors and members of the public who might be affected by their activities. The most recent advance in that process has been in response to a major European 'framework' Directive, with five 'daughters', which have been implemented in the UK as a set of Regulations associated with the Management of Health and Safety at Work Regulations 1992. They are more explicit on the need to identify, remove or control hazards.

Box 10.3: Occupational health legislation

- Management of Health and Safety at Work Regulations 1992

- Provision and Use of Work Equipment Regulations 1992

- Personal Protective Equipment at Work Regulations 1992

- Manual Handling Operations Regulations 1992

- Workplace (Health Safety and Welfare) Regulations 1992

- Health and Safety (Display Screen Equipment) Regulations 1992

Synopsis of health and safety obligations

There are many other health, safety and welfare regulations affecting the health sector of industry, including general practice itself. In this complex and wide ranging legislation, the concept of risk is of particular importance.

Hazards, which remain potential until they cause harm, may be physical, chemical, mechanical or biological. Psychological hazards have long been recognised in the organisation and in systems of work.

Risk represents the probability of a hazard causing harm or damage to people, plant or premises. A sequence of steps first embodied in the Control of Substances Hazardous to Health (COSHH) Regulations 1988 are now applied to the identification and control of any risks at the place of work. The best available technology not entailing excessive cost must be used to achieve that end.

Risk assessment and control

All employers must carry out a competent, suitable and sufficient assessment of the activities in which they are engaged to identify such risks. The assessment must be recorded, if only to indicate that no risk is perceived. Any persons providing employers with health and safety assistance are expected to be competent to do so.

Identified risks must be eliminated if reasonably practicable, if not, they must be reduced and adequately controlled by appropriate means.

This control of risks from a wide variety of hazards must be measured to ensure that it is effective. If there is any doubt of the complete control of a hazard, or if the measuring instrument is not sufficiently sensitive, initial and periodic biological measurement of the worker may be necessary to ensure that the hazard is having no perceptible effect.

There must also be compliance in one's own practice. The hazards of body fluids are within the scope of the COSHH Regulations. The risk of hepatitis B infection of health care workers or patients has since been competently assessed in detail in medical literature and in a wide variety of publications by the DoH, the BMA and other professional bodies. That documentation quantifies the risk, identifies those employees and patients (members of the public) exposed to it and sets out standards of adequate control. Despite the passage of five years, many employers in the public and private health sectors have not taken more than the first step in protecting employees, contractors or members of the public. Many individual employees and contractors appear innocent or even ignorant of the risk of either infection or criminal prosecution for failing to take adequate action.

Fitness for the job

Health surveillance and medical examinations are therefore neither the major component of occupational health nor the major need of the working population. At engagement, the vast majority of the working population select themselves effectively by choosing from the jobs available the one best suited to their individual needs and capabilities. In clerical and retail occupations, the 'medical' component of the selection procedure may be performed by the engaging manager without intrusion into privacy.

Box 10.4: Factors in health surveillance

- A previous history is the most reliable predictor of back trouble in the future.

- Reference of a good attendance record with the previous employer or educator is the most reliable predictor of future satisfactory attendance.

- The history of previous employment is an indicator of the probability of noise-induced hearing loss.

- Binocular vision is most easily tested by the reading of a motor vehicle number plate. (It is negligent to allow monocular vision to be put at risk.)

Health screening

Medical examination itself has no preventive function. The needs for, and the standards of, initial and subsequent health assessments are set out in the HSE guidance notes on pre-employment screening and health surveillance by routine procedures. Complexity ranges from self-reporting by the trained employee, to full examination with laboratory and other investigations.

Health questionnaire

At initial engagement, a self-completed health questionnaire may be an adequate screening mechanism. Nursing or medical staff are required to interpret confidential clinical information in the replies to a health questionnaire into staffing terms. The most comprehensive questionnaires allow periodic repetition to include health and life-style promotion measures. Periodic routine screening is intended to detect abnormality at the earliest stage, so that exposure may be stopped or necessary treatment begun as soon as possible. Protocols must therefore use state-of-the-art technology, standardise the conditions of each test for all subjects and repeat tests in the same conditions, if they are to be consistent when viewed as a series.

Common surveillance procedures

In relation to some hazardous occupations, programmes of specific tests have long been set out in statute. Examples include those for lead workers, and people working with carcinogenic substances or ionising radiations, and with compressed air.

Box 10.5: Diagnostic surveillance procedures

- Blood estimations are usually related to acute or chronic exposure to chemicals.

- Lung function tests detect acute or chronic spasm in asthma, or scarring of lung tissue due to chronic inflammatory disease.

- Chest X-rays show the deposition of minerals or the effects of acute or chronic inflammation of the lung.

- Audiometry (a soundproof booth is essential) may be a defence in litigation.

Confidentiality

Health surveillance records have two components. Clinical detail is subject to medical confidentiality in a medical record. The health record is open to management, so that appropriate steps may be taken to remove an individual from further exposure if necessary. If a health record is required (eg immunisation status or level of lead in blood) to be raised, it may have to be retained for subsequent inspection for years (in some cases, at least 30 years).

Environmental records

Health records are of little value unless related to accurate contemporary records of the environment, since the cause of change can only be identified as being inside the work-place if the interior environment is known.

Opportunities

The total workforce of 26 million in the UK is distributed in comparatively small groups, 90% of them numbering 25 workers or less. The pattern of employment in which workers are widely dispersed means that those in small groups are frequently those at greatest risk. Fewer than half of all employers are aware of health and safety issues. In manufacturing industries, only about 15% of companies provide anything more than first aid cover at the place of work. Slightly more than 1000 full-time occupational physicians of consultant status care for their workers. In this, they are assisted by about 2500 doctors working part time in occupational medicine, most of whom are GPs with no formal qualification in occupational medicine. There are some 5000 estimated nurses working in occupational medicine in private sector companies, most of whom hold an occupational health nursing certificate. Some are distributed in larger commercial organisations, in occupational health departments containing the usual hierarchy of doctors, nurses and other disciplines. More frequently, a nurse works entirely alone, perhaps with the occasional help of a part-time occupational health physician. While, in such circumstances, the doctor will always be ultimately accountable for clinical matters, the nurse employed by the company may be responsible for managing its service.

The programme for action of *The Health of the Nation*, and the developments described in general legislation, as they might affect the NHS in particular, may stimulate an increase in the demand for expertise in occupational medicine. However, the reaction is severely constrained by the economic climate, especially as it affects health authorities, NHS Trusts and general practices working within fixed budgets.

In 1994, the NHS Executive issued Health Service Guidelines HSG(94)51, *Occupational health services of NHS staff*, which sets out the statutory framework that must be reflected in the health and safety policy. An occupational health service should now be regarded as a formal arrangement for the implementation of that policy. The Guidelines indicate that managers should ensure that every occupational health team has access to, and advice from, a consultant occupational physician, as required. When the occupational health service of the NHS Trust has achieved its own purpose, it might then be in a position to make available that consultant expertise to outside organisations as readily as is now the case in virtually every other clinical speciality.

Responsibility to employer and employee

The relationship between the employer and the doctor is complex. In negotiating the contract, the doctor must make it clear that advice will be impartial, and that the relationships with the employees on clinical matters will be subject to medical confidentiality. The Faculty of Occupational Medicine, Royal College of Physicians, has published *Guidance on Ethics for Occupational Physicians*, which outlines many of the particular problems encountered in the practice of occupational medicine. The BMA booklet *The Occupational Physician* describes, in broad terms, the role of the doctor working in service or production industries in the public and private sectors. An annual supplement on suggested fees is provided free to BMA members.

Absence control

While the benefits of an occupational health service may be attractive in their own right, nearly every employer who provides one expects the potential benefits of lower sickness absence, increased productivity and reduced turnover. In this respect, the doctor in industry has as an ultimate objective the profitability of the operation. The GP practising at the place of work is likely to be caring in that role for patients of other colleagues' neighbouring practices, and will probably meet some patients of the home practice as employees. The most likely conflict of interest is in relation to the control of absence behaviour. A sick pay policy should seek to protect the employee from loss of earnings during illness. In return, the employee is generally expected to observe discipline in notifying absence in good time. Good employers will help in rehabilitation and redeployment, and all wish to direct benefit to those who are ill. Absence attributed to sickness may be due to a disability that causes continuous absence of several weeks. Repeated short period claims are a separate phenomenon, in that while there may be a medical component, absence is generally provoked by a number of other issues to do with motivation, the nature of the job and the quality of management. The Arbitration Conciliation and Advisory Service (ACAS) has published a booklet on *Absence*, which sets out these factors in some detail, and they are summarised in the booklet '*Administration of Statutory Sick Pay* published by the DSS.

Should an employee be unable to contribute to the needs of the business, service may be terminated even in the presence of incapacity. However, an industrial tribunal will expect the employer to be able to demonstrate that the decision was not precipitate, that medical advice was sought on behalf of the employers that the employee's doctor had an opportunity to comment, and that the employee had been made aware of the impact of the pattern of absence on the conduct of business in the department.

An occupational physician may be asked to make formal medical enquiries, while satisfying the requirements of the Access to Medical Reports Act. The medical enquiry is intended to provide information to improve the quality of a management decision.

Box 10.6: Management of sickness and ill-health

The manager requires from the doctor the answers to the following questions:

- What is the likely date of return to work?

- Will there be any disability at that time?

- Will it be temporary or permanent?

- Is there an underlying, remediable cause for the pattern of absence?

- Is there a likelihood of regular and efficient service in the future?

It is the occupational physician's job to interpret the clinical situation of the employee/patient to give answers to those questions. The timescale is entirely different from that of those providing therapy. Clinically, there may be some evidence of progress not amounting to complete recovery. It is perfectly legitimate for a clinician to defer a final judgement, perhaps for months. This is an entirely unrealistic timescale for a manager trying to provide a service or to produce goods each day. The occupational physician therefore has to make a definite prediction and to answer the above questions within a timescale of three weeks, the limit set in the Access to Medical Reports Act.

To act as therapist for one's own patient, while advising the employer upon the likelihood of that individual being able to continue to work regularly and effectively, is a conflict of interest that is extremely difficult to resolve. The most careful record of a full explanation of the purpose and possible outcome of the medical report is essential. The article 'Statutory sick pay' in *Occupational Health Review*, (June/July issue 1986) may be a helpful guide.

The Access to Medical Reports Act certainly applies to a doctor in a therapeutic relationship with an individual. It would seem that it may not embrace those records kept by an occupational physician, although this has not yet been tested in law.

Organisations

The medical division of the HSE which enforces legislation also publishes documents on many aspects of health and safety, in particular a medical series of guidance notes on a wide range of occupational medical topics.

The Faculty of Occupational Medicine sets and maintains standards of excellence. The Society of Occupational Medicine has a wide membership requiring no special qualification. It is organised in a number of provinces throughout the UK. It arranges evening meetings on various topics of interest for occupational physicians and holds an annual scientific meeting. The Occupational Health Committee of the BMA is concerned primarily with terms and conditions of service, but advises the profession as a whole on topics concerned with health and safety legislation. The Association of National Health Service Occupational Physicians is perhaps the largest special interest group for occupational physicians. There is also a Section of Occupational Medicine in the Royal Society of Medicine.

The recent reorganisation of general practice in the NHS may alter the pattern of part-time GP participation in occupational medicine. Until recently, members of a practice might carry out an occasional session during the week as private practice. The recent alteration in the contract for general medical services may inhibit that trend. Sessions may no longer be feasible if the minimum commitment to general medical services is to be observed.

Qualifications and training

In large organisations, the major health and safety resources for management are the doctor, the nurse, the hygienist and the safety officer. Standards of competence have been set for each of these disciplines. While many large organisations will employ an occupational hygienist, or use other experts within the business to carry out similar functions, smaller employers may expect the doctor to give advice on the working environment. Occupational medicine is practised in a multidisciplinary field, requiring knowledge of complex health, safety and employment legislation. The Faculty of Occupational Medicine has set out in detail the requirements of a Diploma in Occupational Medicine and for associateship and membership of the Faculty. The range of qualifications allows for part-time study. The Society of Occupational Medicine organises frequent local evening meetings on specific topics in occupational health. The Institute of Occupational Medicine, University of Birmingham, and the Departments of Occupational Medicine of the Universities of Edinburgh and Manchester, provide training, and there is a distance learning course of reading, audio- and videotapes available from the University of Manchester.

Further reading

1   The Faculty of Occupational Medicine of the Royal College of Physicians has produced a second edition of *Fitness for Work* (Oxford Medical Publications, Oxford).
2   NHS Executive Letter HSG(94)51, 6 December 1994, has appendices setting out lists of health and safety legislation and of professional bodies.
3   The BMA publishes *The Occupational Physician*, which is a summary of the role. An annual supplement on suggested pay scales is available, free of charge to members, from local BMA offices.

11　Sports medicine

Stuart Carne

One morning, about 35 years ago, I received a letter out of the blue (if you'll forgive the pun), from Alec Stock, the then manager of Queen's Park Rangers Football Club, inviting me to meet him to discuss the medical arrangements at the club.[a] Their previous medical officer had retired after nearly 30 years service with the club, and they were looking for a successor: was I interested? I was very interested. Now that I was too old to play, it would be a way for me still to be involved in one of my favourite relaxations.

How do clubs identify their possible club doctor? There were – and still are – no lists of approved sports medical officers. What happened in my case was much more basic. The chap who made the directors' tea and poured the whisky after the match was my patient. He heard them talking about their need for a doctor. His doctor, he told them, was a keen soccer fan, and from that small acorn grew my extra role for over 30 years as medical officer to what is now a successful soccer team in the Premier League. When I retired from ordinary practice, the club made me their Vice President, so I retain my connections.

The title Honorary Medical Officer is still bestowed on most sports club doctors, and is, in fact very close to the truth; indeed, it is often the whole truth, for most medical officers to professional sports clubs are paid only a small honorarium. Medical officers to amateur clubs are usually paid nothing at all. This applies in most sports, including both ball games and athletics.

Some individuals who are 'giants' in their sport may have their own personal physician, but that is exceptional. In most cases, anyway, only the official medical officer is allowed in the dressing room.

GP or specialist?

GPs who practise sports medicine should remember the limitations of their

---

[a]Queen's Park Rangers play in blue and white hoops.

expertise and not attempt to undertake treatments for which they do not possess the necessary skills. In the context of medical negligence, doctors may be judged not only on the standards expected of average practitioners in their branch of the profession, but also on the standards of care expected from other doctors offering that particular service. Therefore the standard of care expected of GPs will normally be judged against the standard of care expected of an average GP; if GPs offer a service that would normally be assumed to fall within the province of a specialist, a court may well judge them by the standard of care expected of a specialist and not that expected of a GP.

Access to specialists who have expertise in sports injuries is crucial. Equally important is their availability. As many sports injuries happen during 'unsocial hours' (weekends and/or evenings), when NHS consultants are not always immediately available, many professional sports clubs also have an honorary orthopaedic consultant. Some clubs have an orthopaedic consultant as their club doctor. As GPs, it is important that we persuade those clubs that do this that they also need a GP: primary care problems are, in my experience, far more numerous than those requiring a specialist, and are better dealt with by an experienced primary care specialist (i.e. a GP).

Consultant advice may also be necessary on non-orthopaedic problems, for example the significance or otherwise of a heart murmur, with particular reference to its influence or otherwise on an athlete's fitness. (It should be noted that abnormal ECGs are frequently found during or immediately after a period of heavy training and are usually of no significance. Similarly, proteinuria – and even haematuria – may be found and does not necessarily signify any renal pathology.)

The role of a GP in sports medicine

Most GPs who are involved in sports medicine do so as a club doctor and/or offer their expertise to sports men and women who have no direct access to a club doctor. A few work at special sports centres, where they sometimes describe themselves as 'specialists in sports medicine' (In the UK, the term 'specialist' is generally held to be synonymous with 'consultant'. The author has, therefore, always described himself as 'a GP with a special interest'.)

GPs normally provide primary sports medical care, which includes:

- assessment of the individual's fitness to train and perform

- advice on how to improve fitness

- the diagnosis and treatment of acute injuries

- advice on how best to recover after an illness or accident.

In addition, a sports medical officer will often be expected to advise on general medical problems, both acute and chronic, particularly if they affect performance.

Emotional problems abound. Some individuals become frustrated when their performance at whatever sporting activity they have chosen fails to match their expectations. They may transfer the blame on to some physical defect or injury – real or imagined – magnifying the 'disability' out of all proportion. A number lack the mental ruggedness needed to achieve maximum performance whenever it is required. A few athletes seem to acquire an injury every time they face a major event. A trained generalist, accustomed to sorting out the physical, social and psychiatric components of ordinary people's illnesses, will find that skill very useful when advising sports men and women.

The duties of a club doctor also include the organisation of a prophylactic immunisation service. In addition, a travel prophylactic service will be necessary for those clubs or individuals needing to travel overseas. The club doctor should supervise all the necessary travel prophylactics as well as giving advice on diet and 'non-sports recreation'.

In some sports, certain specific requirements for medical care are laid down by the governing body of that sport. For example, in horse racing, appointed doctors have to be available *at the course* on every race day. Similarly, a doctor has to be present at every major soccer and rugby match – and that means being at the ground throughout the match, and not just on call. (In the UK, the person who runs onto the pitch when someone is injured at a soccer match is usually the club physiotherapist. In many other countries, the doctor also runs on to the pitch; indeed, some Italian clubs seem to have at least two doctors for every injury!)

At major sports events, notably premier league soccer, rugby (both union and league), boxing and horse racing, it is now necessary for a doctor, with full ambulance and possibly paramedical back-up, to be available *on site* to cope with accidents and illnesses among the spectators. It will normally be necessary for a doctor other than the club doctor to take on this role. Although a number of GPs are employed in this capacity, many clubs prefer to rely on the local accident and emergency consultant (where one is available) to organise this aspect of their medical responsibilities.

Training

There are now a number of courses for doctors wanting to be involved in sports medicine, but there are, at present, no official standards for training. A working party has been set up by the Royal Medical Colleges (including the RCGP), in collaboration with the major sports medical associations, to look at the possibility of setting up an inter-collegiate faculty of sports medicine. It is hoped that, in future, any doctor who takes up sports medicine will have had adequate training and possess an appropriate qualification.

Relationships with other GPs

A sports club doctor is somewhat akin to an occupational health physician. The rules that apply to the relationship between an occupational health physician and the patient's GP therefore also apply to sports medicine, although there are, in practice, significant differences. It is, therefore, absolutely essential for a GP who is acting as a club doctor to remember that the sports person will almost certainly have his or her own GP.

The patient and, for that matter, the club do not see the issue in the same light. Not infrequently, professional sports people will have had little personal contact with a GP since childhood. They therefore see no reason why the club doctor should not take on that role. However, club doctors have to remember that, if they are to be the GP as well, they must be available at all times – including nights and weekends – to make house calls when asked. This may not be possible, however willing the doctor may be, when the athlete lives 20 miles or more away from the club, as, for example, many London footballers do.

It is therefore essential for the club doctor to maintain contact with the patient's GP and seek his permission, *in advance* whenever possible, to initiate treatment and/or specialist referral.

Relationships with other professionals

Physiotherapists

Many professional sports clubs now employ their own *full-time* physiotherapist. Because the physiotherapist is generally on site, he or she will often form a relationship with the players that is much closer than that of the club doctor, who is likely to be available only once or twice a week (plus match days). The club doctor must therefore be able to work in harmony with the physiotherapist. Nowadays, physiotherapists do not take 'instructions' from the doctor: they are fully trained professionals in their own right. Any differences of opinion about how certain injuries should be managed need, therefore, to be ironed out in advance.

Osteopaths

Many athletes find that osteopathic treatment is often helpful in getting them fit again, and a number prefer osteopathy to orthodox medicine. A medical qualification offers no special privileges in that respect. In today's world, consumer choice rules, and *caveat emptor* can apply as much to the doctor as it does to the alternative practitioner. It need not be too difficult for the club doctor and the osteopath to respect one anothers' skills without coming into conflict or denying the other's professional status.

NHS or private?

There is no reason why athletes should be given priority when they want a specialist appointment at an NHS hospital. In the past, it may have been possible to queue-jump, but this is now both rare and difficult at most hospitals.

Professional athletes, like professional performers in fields, such as dance, music and theatre, want their medical problems dealt with quickly. A professional footballer is not willing to miss a dozen – or even only three or four – matches while he is waiting for an outpatient appointment to see a specialist. For that reason, many professional sports clubs take out private medical insurance.

It must be remembered, however, that this does *not* cover any fees that a GP might wish to charge. Furthermore, unless the person being treated is on the GP's NHS list of patients, any medicine required must be prescribed on a private prescription. (Writing private prescriptions also has an educational component: it teaches us the cost of many of the drugs we would normally prescribe and helps us to identify cheaper and equally satisfactory alternatives.)

Fees

As there are no agreed fees for GPs involved in sports medicine, doctors need to negotiate an appropriate professional fee with an event's organiser, for example a boxing promoter, or with a football club's management. The BMA produces guidance to doctors attending sporting events, as well as an hourly professional rate. Members can, however, seek further information from their **local** BMA office.

Many sports clubs – especially amateur clubs – are themselves under enormous financial constraints and are not able to afford anything resembling the fee the doctor might expect for the time and expertise put in; indeed, many say they are unable to pay any fee at all and rely on the goodwill (and keenness) of the doctor. Even some wealthy sports clubs often baulk at the idea of paying a doctor what is, by any standard, a very modest fee. (It is highly unlikely that the club doctor asked to assess the fitness of a £5 million footballer will be paid anything over and above the normal annual retainer.)

Some clubs pay an annual retainer for which they expect *total* cover. The sports club doctor who is not available on every match day, or who cannot provide a suitable deputy is of little use to the club. GPs appointed to this work will therefore have to make arrangements within the practice to ensure their availability to the club. In some sports, for example tennis and horse racing, the need for medical cover is concentrated into two or three weeks a year, during which time the doctors will find they have little or no time for anything else in the practice (or at home), and may well feel they need a holiday afterwards to recuperate. In such cases, it is not unreasonable for the doctors to expect to be reimbursed for at least the cost of a locum in the practice, but, again, this usually has to be left to individual negotiation.

Some clubs and sports associations recognise this problem and offer an adequate fee as well as expenses. Others believe that a free seat in the grandstand for the doctor and (*perhaps*), for a spouse, plus a cup of tea, is adequate remuneration. Notwithstanding, the situation has improved, and medical advisers to professional sports clubs should no longer be out of pocket. GPs who undertake this work should not expect to get rich financially, but most sports doctors, nevertheless, seem to derive great pleasure from their involvement – and no fee can substitute for the thrill when your club wins a major trophy.

12　Surgical work in general practice

Brian Elvy

Prior to the reforms of recent years, GPs performing surgical work outside their own practice population were a rarity. Health authorities did not place work outside their directly managed units, and local private units employed only specialist surgeons. Indeed, most referring GPs would have been uneasy about such a development. With purchaser/provider separation, purchasers, such as GP fundholders and health authorities (or commissions), are now not only able to consider placing work with other providers, but are also actively being encouraged to manage a shift towards primary care level wherever and whenever possible. It is important to understand that we are therefore discussing GPs in the performance of surgical work as *independent providers* and not as employees of, for example, NHS Trusts or private units. It is also important to understand that this work is *still for the NHS* but out-with general medical services. It represents an opportunity for appropriately trained and motivated GPs to generate income. However, opportunities for surgical work entirely outside the NHS are likely to remain limited. Notwithstanding the title of this book, it is nevertheless a new potential for additional employment and income for many GPs.

These developments are not designed to encourage *all* GPs to do surgical work, but rather to make it possible for purchasers to engage those with appropriate skills. The attraction to purchasers is that, with low overheads, most GPs can perform work at a lower unit cost, more quickly and in more patient-friendly surroundings. The attraction to the GP provider is that of income generation and professional development and satisfaction.

This chapter outlines how an interested and able GP can achieve the goal of becoming a provider of surgical services. While it will be assumed that such contracts will be for minor surgery, there is no reason in principle why any GP trained to a higher surgical standard should not seek and secure a contract for any surgical service, providing he or she can satisfy a purchaser of his or her ability to deliver work to an agreed standard of quality and quantity.

The issue of surgical provision by a fundholder to his own patients is separate (although parallel). Some of the hurdles to approval, however, are identical.

What is involved?

The number of stages required to secure a provider contract might seem daunting, particularly, perhaps, to a non-fundholder, who may not be so familiar with the contracting process as are his fundholding colleagues. However, the potential GP surgeon can be reassured that he need only apply those negotiation and management skills that he uses to provide his or her general medical services. It is also essential to have an efficient practice manager who is knowledgeable in contract negotiation and running the system.

Box 12.1: Contracting for private minor surgery

The first steps in securing a provider contract are:

- outline a plan of intended service

- outline an agreement with partners

- make the initial approach to purchaser(s)

- begin contract negotiations.

The potential GP surgeon will have already been thinking of providing a service to a potential purchaser (or purchasers), so, having verified that he or she can satisfy the broad requirements, an initial approach is made. At the same time, purchasers will be seeking potential alternative providers, although some initial inertia of established custom and practice may need to be overcome. For many purchasers, this will be breaking new ground and may be perceived as a risk. The budding provider should sell himself with confidence.

There will be a need early on to agree with partners issues such as readjustment of general medical services work-load, division of income, medico-legal anxieties and postoperative responsibility. The work-load of practice staff will need to be planned in outline. Much will depend on such variables as practice agreements, systems of profit sharing, other outside commitments, fundholding, etc. It is unlikely that a well-run practice with good supporting management will have problems, but any variations in the partnership agreement should be conducted in the usual way.

Having reached the stage of serious negotiation with purchasers, the detailed requirements are thereafter covered by considering the contracting process.

The contracting process

Box 12.2 covers the main areas for consideration. Standard purchaser/provider contracts can be used with customised 'fine-tuning' applied. Most purchasers will have them ready prepared.

Box 12.2: Key contract issues

- Choose cost per case contracts
- Performance targets
- Price per case
- Payment arrangements
- Contract period
- Annual review and contract renewal
- Quality standards
- Appointment system
- Arbitration arrangements
- Variation arrangements
- *Force majeure*
- Subcontracting arrangements
- Relevant legislation
- Confidentiality
- Indemnity

The initial negotiation takes place by exchange of letters, but final agreements are reached after one or more contract meetings. It should be remembered that contract negotiation is a two-way process and needs to be approached flexibly by both sides. The final result is a series of mutually agreed compromises. The intended provider must be prepared for detailed examination of his or her arrangements, and to adjust to the purchaser's needs.

Performance targets

The purchaser will set out what is required. This may be a specified number of surgical events or a set budget, or both. The purchaser may wish to place the whole contract with one provider or to divide it between two or more. The attraction of the latter approach is one of insurance against lost production should a provider fall by the wayside. The provider should take what is on offer, although any ambition to expand, accompanied by evidence of output capability, should be made plain at an early stage of contract renewal. This will require a good business plan.

Pricing and contract type

The potential provider's prices will need to be competitive. Where the alternative is an NHS Trust, there should not be a problem for the provider, because his overheads and intended profit margin will be lower. When competing with other GP providers, securing the contract is likely to be more difficult, and contract sharing may be an option that needs to be considered.

There are three contract types in common use: block, cost and volume, and cost per case. Cost per case is to be recommended, although the purchaser may set a ceiling on activity with a fixed budget. The contract period is often one year, although provision for roll-over, year-on-year contracts should be negotiated. Payment should be monthly in arrears, with an agreed deadline, and penalties for late payment should be included.

Appointment systems and waiting lists

The purchaser will wish to contract responsibility for both these functions. Costings will need to include this, and software packages are easily obtained to create one's own system.

In these early days of shifting work from traditional hospital-based providers, there have been examples of resistance by NHS Trusts. For example, where a waiting list is being transferred, this has on occasions been stalled by the refusal of hospital clinicians to hand over patient details, and the withholding of referral letters. This is the responsibility of the purchaser, who may have to exert pressure for their release or obtain replacements or copies. With time, it is hoped that these tactics will disappear. The provider should not involve himself in disputes of this nature.

Quality standards

This is the most important section in a contract. While contract-shifting remains a sensitive area, both parties will be keen to demonstrate to any critics that the service they intend to produce will be equal or superior to that which existed before. Close attention to all the points in Box 12.3 is essential as all contracts will contain a series of quality assurance clauses covering the following areas.

Box 12.3: Quality issues

- Relevant Charter standards

- Information for patients

- Follow-up arrangements

- Waiting list management

- Maximum waiting times

- Performance review

- Audit and value for money

- Patient feedback

- Complaints

- Premises and equipment

- Staff training

- Resuscitation arrangements

Premises

For minor surgery, a sterile operating room is not essential, but the standard of cleanliness must be high. Nursing staff must be trained in control of infection procedures, and cleaning staff must be instructed in room-cleaning procedures. Work surfaces should be clear of clutter that may attract dust or deter efficient cleaning. An overhead extractor fan is desirable but not essential, unless contracted for.

If the GP's premises are subject to cost-rent it is essential that he or she checks with the FHSA that gross income does not infringe the 10% rule.

Equipment and clothing

A potential provider must acquire all necessary equipment, including surgical instruments, hyfrecators, cryosprays and cautery machines, plus surgical gowns and gloves. He must also provide adequate means of sterilisation. Whether this be by the GP's own steriliser (of an acceptable model, adequately and regularly maintained and certified) or by local CSSD supply will be a matter for choice, and costed accordingly. The potential purchaser may well, and probably should, wish to include a clause allowing inspection of equipment and premises at any time. If the purchaser wishes to stipulate types of equipment for the service, there may have to be negotiation on this.

Resuscitation

Provision of resuscitation equipment will be important and the purchaser may wish to stipulate that staff undergo regular training. For local anaesthetic procedures, this need be no more than that required for general medical services purposes. If, however, general anaesthetic procedures are proposed, the standard of resuscitation may need to be appropriately higher.

Techniques

These are a matter of clinical judgement and should not ordinarily concern the purchaser. However, the provider may need to demonstrate competence in an appropriate range of techniques to his or her purchasers. It should be ensured that the contract states which techniques or skills are being purchased and which are not. It is always worth remembering the maxim – if in doubt, put it in the contract.

Pre- and post-operative communication

Over the years, the medical profession has been criticised for poor communication with patients, particularly in providing adequate information before and after procedures. More recently, there have been moves to address this weakness, and there are now many good examples of information 'hard copy' that can be sent or given to patients before, during and after medical events. The prospective provider must expect a clause in his contract requiring this to be done in all cases, ideally in the form of information leaflets.

Follow-up

Anyone conducting surgical procedures must expect post-operative complications despite the maintenance of high standards, and the provider may be contracted to provide a follow-up service. For minor surgical procedures, follow-up should be infrequent and, in the main, will consist simply of reassurance and advice. The practice will need to discuss how this is delegated during off-duty times. In the event of partners not being willing or able to share such a responsibility, the contract should say so, and in this case, responsibility, in the surgeon's absence will revert in the usual way to the patient's own GP.

Patient satisfaction feedback and audit

These requirements are now standard in any service contract. For minor surgery, simple systems should suffice. Feedback from patients need only be a simple questionnaire presented at the time of operation for return by an agreed date, for example one month post-operatively. Audits of performance activity, complication rates and any other quality criteria can be conducted from these and other data, and a member of the practice staff should be delegated to do the 'number-crunching' for in-year monitoring and annual reports.

Other contract issues

All standard contracts will contain sections on such issues as contract monitoring arrangements, in-year performance reviews, variation (i.e. significant changes to the terms of the contract within year), subcontracting, confidentiality, arbitration, complaints arrangements, *force majeure* (i.e. what to do if unforseeable events should render the contract unviable for either party) and value-for-money and efficiency conditions. While this list may seem daunting or even boring to the budding surgeon-provider, he or she must develop an acquaintance with them and discuss their negotiation with the practice manager. For this kind of contract, they are actually quite simple to arrange. Health authorities or commissions tend to produce very detailed contracts, but this will hopefully improve with time. Fundholders are generally happy to set much simpler contracts.

Patient's Charter

Box 12.4: Patient's Charter

- equity
- effectiveness
- accessibility
- appropriateness
- responsiveness.

As a provider of secondary care, relevant Charter standards will apply to the GP surgeon. All purchasers, fundholders and health commissions alike will contract for these, using local as well as national standards. The responsibility for their audit will be with the provider, for presentation at agreed intervals. The relatively small sise of any one GP provider's scale of activity should ensure that none of these presents a problem. In addition, in the author's opinion, a number of the standard Charter criteria will be irrelevant, so it is suggested time is spent negotiating an agreement with the purchaser on what standards are and are not to be applied. Remember – if in doubt, put it in the contract.

Training and experience

Prospective purchasers will want to check the level of experience and expertise of any future provider. The most likely route to the required skills will be through some sort of basic and/or further training within the secondary sector, starting with the junior ranges of surgical firms, and possibly clinical assistant, hospital practitioner or even associate specialist grades. Some practitioners might have postgraduate surgical qualifications that were acquired before settling to a general practice career.

There are other sources of training and experience available that would be acceptable to purchasers. For example, the Marie Stopes organisation will provide training in vasectomy. A 'virgin' surgeon, having completed appropriate training and presented a business plan, might be able to negotiate a contract, although, in this situation, a prudent purchaser would probably seek a trial period and frequent appraisal.

It is *not* a requirement, however, for the GP surgeon to have a postgraduate surgical degree.

Medical indemnity

The defence societies apply a scale of differential subscriptions based on actuarial assessment of the likely risk of litigation, for example, the rate for a GP is much lower than for a plastic surgeon.

At the time of writing, the defence societies have no plans to load the subscriptions of GP minor surgeons, although they are aware of developments and may move from this stance in the future, depending on any eventual increase in litigation from this direction. The Medical Protection Society has stated that, in its case, standard insurance covers operations conducted under local anaesthetic. If a practitioner is using a general anaesthetic, the Society reserves the right to adjust the subscription. These guidelines apply irrespective of the actual volume of surgical work undertaken. It is advisable, therefore, to consult one's defence society when developing plans for service provision, as any such increase would have to be included in costings. Many feel that there should be a clause in the contract to cover this issue, but not all purchasers insist on it.

The future

Crystal ball-gazing is always tempting, so to finish this chapter a few thoughts on the future are offered. If we accept the present government's determination to promote primary care-led purchasing (through the spread of fundholding, and its pressure on health authorities and commissions to seek the views of non-fundholders for their own purchasing processes), and if we accept that many of these purchasers will be seeking alternative provision of a number of services (using such criteria as cost, speed, the provision of service closer to patients' homes etc), it seems reasonable to expect that, with time, the provision of minor surgical work by GPs will increase. To start with, this increase is likely to be slow but steady, while confidence is gained on both sides, and the early pioneers must be, in a sense, ambassadors for those coming after them. The ground rules for such services must be firmly set and strictly followed to protect against the potential for criticism that such services are second best or of a low standard. The early participants must be prepared to become involved in setting these frameworks and, possibly, also policing them.

A change of government could, of course, bring a change of emphasis or even a major change of policy. This would mean a potential long-term investment risk for GP surgeons. Many feel, however, that the provider/purchaser split is here to stay, so, providing GP surgeons establish beyond doubt the reputation of their services for reliability and value for money, no government would wish to return to a more costly and slower service.

Old moulds have been broken, and innovative and entrepreneurial instincts can now be followed by those who wish to use them. To that extent, at least, we are perhaps seeing the return of an earlier GP spirit. *Plus ça change . . .*, and happy negotiating.

References

1   NHS Executive (1994) *The operation of the NHS internal market.* HSG(94)55.
2   NHS Executive (1993) GP *fundholding practices: the provision of secondary care.* HSG(93)14.
3   East Norfolk Health Commission (unpublished) *Managing the shift* (draft document).
4   Service contract between East Norfolk Health Authority and Oak Street Medical Practice, Norwich 1994/5.

13 Doctors, solicitors and the courts: a guide to accepting and receiving instructions

Angela Anstey

Doctors are often approached by solicitors on behalf of their clients and requested to provide a medical report for the purposes of legal proceedings. These requests can arise out of a variety of circumstances, and the reason for the request may not be immediately clear to the doctor concerned. It may be that the doctor has already attended the patient in the course of his employment, for example in the accident and emergency department, the injuries for which the patient was then treated are the subject of a police investigation or a civil claim for damages, and the only person who is qualified to comment on the nature and extent of the injuries is in fact the doctor who dealt with the original incident and who had no knowledge of the circumstances. Alternatively, the doctor may have witnessed a bank robbery and may be a valuable witness for the prosecution or the defence. In some situations, he may even be the leading expert in his field whose expertise will be invaluable to the case of the patient/client.

When a doctor is first approached to act in a case, he should expect to be given clear and concise instructions on what is expected of him in terms of the area of expertise, the nature of the report to be provided, the type of case and full consent from the patient for the release of his medical records, bearing in mind that there is nowadays a tendency for the whole of the patient's medical history to be disclosed at the outset to his medical and legal advisers.

Box 13.1: Checklist of initial information

- Patient's details, including name, address, date of birth and, if possible, telephone number.

- Basic information about who one is acting for, for example the patient or a defendant to a negligence action.

- Whether or not the plaintiff is receiving legal aid.

- Whether or not the proceedings have begun.

- The urgency of the instructions – is there a time problem?

- Valid consent from the patient for the release of his or her medical records.

- If opposed to the patient, his or her consent to be examined by you.

- The particular nature of the expert opinion sought.

- A history of the incident or accident or what, broadly speaking, is the patient's version of events.

Staying involved

Once the patient has been examined and the medical report has been sent off to the instructing solicitor, it is up to the doctor to ensure that he is now prepared to honour his obligations towards the patient. This means that he has accepted a degree of responsibility towards the patient and must ensure that he does not lose sight of this over the next few years or months. It frequently takes much longer for a case to come to court than either the expert or the patient expects, which can cause both of them problems. If a doctor is habitually instructed by the same firm of solicitors, he becomes familiar with the way in which they work and may feel able to ask them what is happening on a particular case or to be updated regularly on the various cases he shares. If he does not feel comfortable asking his instructing solicitor for an update, he may have no idea of the progress of the case and may suddenly be surprised when requested to attend in court for the final trial. He may then feel that he is not adequately prepared, and resent the request. This is clearly not in the patient's best long-term interests, and GPs are therefore advised to write at intervals to the instructing solicitor for a progress report and keep on writing until a reply is received.

What type of witness are you?

A professional person may attend court as a witness in one of three capacities.

- An ordinary witness.

- A professional witness.

- An expert witness.

An ordinary witness

This is a witness who will give evidence to the court on what was seen as an ordinary member of the public, for example the doctor who has witnessed a robbery and has subsequently been called to court to give evidence of identification. Acting in this capacity has nothing to do with one's abilities or skills as a doctor.

A professional witness

This is defined as a witness practising as a member of the legal or medical professions, or as a dentist, a veterinary surgeon or accountant who attends to give professional evidence on matters of fact.

This may include, for example, an accident and emergency officer who may have admitted to hospital a man suffering from a stab wound. As a professional witness, he will be asked details of the identity of the victim, how he got to hospital, what injuries were present, what the man's condition was and where was he sent from the accident and emergency department. He may also be expected to give evidence on what happened to the patient in the end.

An expert witness

This category of witness gives opinion evidence on matters within his personal knowledge and is typically called in by one side or the other to interpret the facts using his expertise. He usually attends voluntarily by accepting the task for a fee, whereas the witnesses to fact in the other two categories have no choice but to attend if the court so requires.

Overlap

These definitions are slightly limited, as a professional witness may become an expert witness even though he had been called for another purpose. For example, the accident and emergency doctor may be the only person in a position to give an opinion on how and by what means the injuries were sustained. Using the same example, if the victim died, a pathologist will be employed specifically to determine and provide evidence and an opinion on the type of knife used, from which direction the blow was struck, and whether or not it could be self-inflicted.

Preparing the report

There is no set format for a medico-legal report, although it has essential elements. A doctor must try to bear in mind exactly what the person instructing him would like to have included in the report, and to remember to keep to his own area of knowledge and experience. He must be careful not to stray into the area of apportioning blame where it would not be appropriate for him to make any such remark.

Box 13.2: Checklist of information to include in a report

- Details such as the date of the examination and of the accident (if appropriate).

- Documentation considered (which records were available).

- Patient's details (name, age, date of birth, marital status, occupation, etc).

- History of the injury, including any current medication.

- Treatment, especially if it is still continuing.

- Present condition (to include mental state if appropriate).

- Effect on life-style.

- Review of clinical data.

- Diagnoses.

- Further treatment, if relevant.

- Prognosis.

- Summary.

Doctors should remember that the patient will see the report, as will the instructing solicitor and possibly the court. It should therefore be concise, clear and easily comprehensible to a non-medical person. If it is easier to describe an injury or complaint in layman's terms by using a diagram, then this should be done. This will make it easier for the court and may well dispose them more favourably to the most concise account, which, of course, guarantees the doctor more instructions in the future.

One should beware of:

- jargon
- irrelevancies
- expressing opinions
- drawing conclusions
- prejudicial comments.

Going to court

Depending on the doctor's relationship with the solicitor who has instructed him, he may receive a varying amount of notice of a hearing date. If the relationship has really broken down, usually owing to a lack of communication, the doctor may find himself in receipt of a witness summons or subpoena to attend court on a date that is either completely new to him or which the solicitor knows is not convenient. It would be contempt of court not to attend, providing the correct expenses have been tendered, so the doctor may find himself having to attempt to repair the damaged relationship in order to appeal to the solicitor's sense of reason. It is often not enough to explain that a doctor has more than one patient, as the solicitor is already aware of that. It could be that the solicitor himself has not been very well prepared and has panicked, believing, because he has not kept the lines of communication open throughout the case, that the witnesses may not be available.

   If there is any doubt at all, it is the responsibility of the doctor to tell those instructing him his usual terms of business and any proposed holiday dates well in advance, especially if he has been notified that the case is likely to be heard that month.

Subpoenas or witness orders

These are orders normally sent through the court to a doctor (witness), requiring him to attend court on a certain dates. Failure to obey these is contempt of court. They are often delivered through the post or by a police officer. They should state on them the name of the accused and the location of the trial. There is often no precise date given, as the case is frequently in what is called a 'warned list', which means that it will start once the previous case has finished, whenever that may be. If a doctor has a problem with the date, he must inform the listing officer of the court as soon as possible and be reasonable about when it would be convenient for him to be there. Just because a holiday has been booked does not necessarily protect it. It has been known for a witness to be compelled to return from honeymoon in order to go to court. Even as a doctor, a sick note from a GP is still required if sickness is a reason why attendance is not possible.

A subpoena is used in civil cases, whereas a witness summons is the appropriate term for criminal cases. Subpoenas, in particular, are being used increasingly by solicitors as a means of protecting themselves from an order for costs being awarded against them personally in the event that a witness fails to attend court.

Penalties for failing to attend

If a witness has failed to attend in court, a warrant for his arrest may be issued to bring him to court. He could then be deemed guilty of contempt of court, which carries various penalties, including a fine and/or imprisonment. This could, in itself, take a doctor into a difficult area, because, if he was attending to give evidence for a patient under his care and failed to attend and was then in contempt of court, he could be brought into professional difficulties with the GMC.

Giving evidence

It is important to remember that all evidence in the English legal system is given under oath, and that a doctor is being called upon as an expert to assist the court in reaching the right decision. He is often there as a professional person, and it is recommended that he should attire himself accordingly, even though he may not anticipate seeing any patients that day. It will help the doctor if he is dressed in a suit, as he will then feel comfortable and feel prepared to be taken seriously. Although this is optional advice, it should definitely be borne in mind. A doctor should attempt to remain impartial at all times and, above all, to keep his head. In some complicated cases, the doctor will be expressing his opinion, in which case it does not matter that not everyone agrees with him. He should not let himself be shaken from his standpoint.

Ten golden rules for giving evidence are:

- speak clearly
- listen to the question
- answer the question
- be brief
- avoid jargon
- know your professional limitation
- admit if you do not know
- keep calm
- disagree without losing your temper
- admit to any mistakes.

The first part of giving evidence in court is to tell the court who one is and what one's qualifications are. This will let the jury and/or the judge know why the doctor is there. This will also help a doctor if he is being taken out of his depth. It is important that a witness remembers the purpose of his attendance and is firm in not being drawn into areas outside his knowledge or expertise. If the answer to a particular question or issue is not known, it is far better to say so than allow oneself to be taken out of the area of expertise or knowledge and then discredited altogether. After all, there may be someone else who has been asked to cover the precise point. If the barrister who is examining or cross-examining the doctor has adopted the tactic of trying to ask questions the doctor has not addressed in his report, the doctor can always appeal to the judge, or whoever is hearing the case, for assistance, by pointing out that he has already said three times that it is not his specialty or field and the line of questioning is still persisting. This should ensure a change of tack.

It is important to remember to address the jury or judge, rather than the person asking the questions. In tribunals, it is especially important to watch the hand of the chairman as he will be taking a long hand note of the evidence. Clear diction is also important.

Giving evidence in court, especially for the first time, can be nerve-racking, so it is important for the witness to be well prepared. All questions must be carefully listened to, and if the question is not phrased so as to be easily comprehensible, to request that it be asked again in a different way – this is perfectly acceptable.

Another sound principle is to remember to answer only the question that is asked and not the question that the doctor either thinks he should have been asked or thought he was being asked. Any time needed for a witness to think of the correct answer or phrasing is permissible, as long as it is not excessive. Witnesses should avoid technical language that has not already been explained to the court, and should not feel embarrassed to use sketches to illustrate a point. However, they should avoid being arrogant or condescending to the barristers or the judge. It helps neither the line of questioning nor the patient's case.

A witness must remember not to let himself, or those instructing him, down by losing his temper. Barristers are trained to catch witnesses out by bringing out inconsistencies and encouraging them to make judgements out of their depth. Do not let them. If the witness does not know the answer, it is important to say so, and the questioning can then move back into areas where he is again qualified to give evidence.

The most important aspect of giving evidence is ensuring that all the facts of the case are to the fore of the mind. Preparation is everything, as doctors will only have one chance to give the evidence, and it must therefore be right first time. It is not sufficient to have read the notes only once, i.e. at the time of the original examination. On the other hand, too much familiarity with the patient could lead a court to feel that the evidence is not as impartial as it should be. It is important to strike a balance. It is also important to have read and discussed the expert report prepared by the other side. As possibly the only doctor there to represent the patient's interest, it is essential to clarify the differences and put all the points as clearly and succinctly as possible. Preparation is obviously the key here.

Personal preparation

There is perhaps nothing worse than arriving late for a hearing and then having to check that all the materials required have arrived with you. It is important as part of the preparation done at home (especially for a doctor who of all the witnesses may have a need to produce a textbook to illustrate his points) that all the materials and diagrams are correctly assembled for the court and that the reports have been read one last time to rehearse the points.

Box 13.3: Checklist for court

- The prepared report and several spare copies.

- The file of the case.

- Any diagrams (or affidavits and exhibits).

- Textbook or reference book.

- Pens and paper.

- Map of the court location.

- Small change for telephone calls.

- Other work to do in case a period of waiting is required (highly likely).

Then:

- Check the transport situation and arrangements.

- Arrive early for the hearing – those instructing you may wish to ask your advice or clarify some point.

- Remind the solicitor of all other commitments if the case looks like overrunning.

- Anticipate nerves and go to the toilet first.

- Ask the court usher to point out the correct court.

One final point before giving evidence is to ask the solicitor instructing the witness how to address the judge or deputy judge who will be hearing the case. A note made on one's hand or a scrap of paper will ensure that his information is not forgotten. A checklist appears below, but it is always best to check additionally with those present on the day in case the arrangements have changed.

Modes of address

- High court – My Lord/My Lady.

- Crown court – Your Honour.

- County court – Your Honour.

- Magistrates' court/stipendiary magistrate – Sir/Madam.

- Chairman of a lay bench – Sir/Madam.

- Coroner's court – Sir/Madam.

- Tribunal chairman – Sir/Madam.

Before leaving court, when a witness has finished giving evidence, it is important that the instructing solicitor is aware that he is about to leave, not because there is a need to discuss money, because this should already have been sorted out, but because, as a matter of formality, the court has to release a witness. This means that he will not be recalled to give any further evidence, and that the day in court is really over.

Experts' meetings

There is one final aspect of being instructed in a case, which ought properly be discussed; the experts' meetings. Before a case goes to trial, an attempt is often made to agree some of the issues to save time and costs. If it is not possible to settle the case in its entirety, the experts are requested to meet, often without their instructing solicitors, to see how far they can agree the outstanding issues between them on the medical evidence. It is vital to remember that nothing should be conceded unless it has been approved by the client, or by the solicitor if the client has instructed him on the point. No careless remarks or admissions should be made, as they could reappear at court to haunt the doctor and be quoted out of context.

Conclusion

Providing a GP has an effective working relationship with the solicitor who instructs him, attending in court should be pleasurable. If the arrangements are made to accommodate the requirements of a GP's job and life-style, it should be an enjoyable way of earning some extra money. If a doctor knows the court system and specialises in the same type of case, even the judges will start to know him, and vice versa. Each doctor should find a method of working and giving evidence that suits him and with which he is comfortable, and he may soon start to gain himself a reputation. He will enjoy a good relationship with other professionals and, hopefully, a successful team.

Further reading

1 Hall JG and Smith GD (1992) *The expert witness*. Barry Rose Law Publishers, Chichester.
2 Knight B (1992) *Legal aspects of medical practice*. Churchill Livingstone, Edinburgh.
3 BMA/Law Society (1992) *Medical evidence: guidance for doctors and lawyers*. BMA/Law Society, London.

14   Medico-legal fees: dealing with solicitors and courts

Frank McKenna

Most GPs will, at some stage of their career, be required to attend court to give evidence. Legal commentators have identified a shift in the attitude of individuals during the last decade towards engaging in litigation in order to pursue claims for issues ranging from injuries sustained in accidents to suing doctors for alleged malpractice or incompetence. As a result of this development, GPs are facing increasing demands on their time from solicitors asking for medical reports so that patients can seek compensation. While medico-legal work can bring welcome financial benefits for GPs, it also offers the prospect of coping with considerable difficulties and inconveniences, for example being served with a subpoena, frustrating delays in receiving payment and cancellation of court hearings without notice. The advice set out in this chapter is intended to offer guidance to GPs involved in medico-legal work. If followed, it should both help to ensure that GPs do not encounter difficulties in dealing with solicitors and offer practical solutions if problems unavoidably occur.

Medical reports produced by GPs may be used in a variety of legal proceedings, including criminal matters (magistrates' or crown court), civil matters (county courts or divisions of the high court) and inquests dealing with deaths (coroner's courts). GPs may be asked to prepare a report based on either the patient's records or a separate examination. Once the report has been sent to the solicitors, a GP may be required to attend court to give evidence in relation to the information contained in his report. The following are examples of situations in which a GP's report may be required.

- The patient is making a claim for medical negligence.

- The report is on the psychiatric state of defendants in criminal proceedings or victims of such proceedings.

- The patient is claiming compensation for an industrial disease, for example asbestosis.

- The patient is claiming damages for injuries sustained in an accident, for example motor vehicle- or work-related.

- The report is in connection with child care case, such as of child abuse.

- The report is for other child care issues, such as adoption, fostering and divorce proceedings.

What to do when contacted by a solicitor

When contacted by a solicitor, it is vital that a GP should ask a number of questions to ensure that he is fully aware of what is being asked of him, as solicitors often complain that a particular report has failed to address fundamental issues relevant to a legal claim or that doctors fail to provide reports in time for legal proceedings.

Box. 14.1: A case taken from BMA files

A firm of solicitors contacted a patient's GP for a detailed medical report. The solicitors did not give specific instructions on the nature of the report, and the GP did not attempt to clarify why the report was required. The patient was not asked to attend an examination prior to producing the report.

Unbeknown to the GP, the patient had been knocked off his bicycle some weeks earlier and had sustained a broken arm as well as minor cuts and bruises. The GP prepared his report, raising issues such as the patient's history of migraine headaches and hypertension, but obviously did not refer to the accident. The solicitors subsequently refused to pay for the report, claiming that it was entirely useless for the legal proceedings intended. After pursuing the matter of non-payment for seven months, the GP accepted the solicitor's offer to pay half of the cost of the original report.

In order to avoid such situations, GPs must clarify what is being required of them. The following questions should suffice for this purpose.

- What kind of report is required? Will it be from examination or notes?

- In what capacity are you being asked to attend court, i.e. professional or expert witness? Most GPs appear as professional witnesses, but some with specialist training, i.e. forensic medical examiners (police surgeons), may be eligible to act as experts (*see* Chapter 13).

- Has the issue of patient consent been satisfactorily addressed?

- What type of proceedings are involved? Criminal or civil? Are you being instructed under the legal aid scheme?

- What is the purpose of the action? What are the details of the incident or injury at issue?

- What precisely are you being asked to do? How soon do they require your report?

What to charge

On the basis of this information, GPs must then tackle the issue of what fees to charge for their professional services. The obligations of NHS GPs are set out in the NHS (General Medical Services) Regulations 1992. The Regulations make it clear that the provision of reports for court cases and attendance at court as a professional witness are not part of an NHS GP's terms of service, and a fee may therefore be claimed. This clarification is important as GPs are increasingly approached by bodies such as local authority social service departments (SSDs) requesting both medical reports and the GP's attendance at a case conference, arguing that GPs must provide these services free of charge as the patient is on their NHS lists. It is worth noting that GPs are only obliged to provide certain *certificates* free of charge to patients or their representatives. In relation to legal matters, Schedule 9 of the terms of service (*see* Chapter 1) only obliges GPs to issue a certificate free of charge to patients who are unfit to attend for jury service.

The fees that GPs may charge for undertaking medico-legal work vary and generally depend on whether or not the solicitor's client is in receipt of legal aid. In legally aided cases, i.e. where the costs are paid by the Legal Aid Board, and those brought by the Crown Prosecution Service (CPS), GPs' fees will be constrained as the costs are met from public finances.

Criminal matters

The CPS, a government department, has responsibility for the prosecution of criminal cases in England and Wales. Up to the point at which investigation ceases, the relevant police authority is responsible for any expenditure involved, including the cost of any medical expertise that may be sought. The BMA has a negotiated agreement with police authorities for these circumstances. Once the investigation is complete, the case is handed over to the CPS, which is then responsible for subsequent expenditure. It is at this stage that most GPs are approached for a detailed medical report. When the CPS commissions the services of a GP to write a report or appear in court, it enters into a contract with the GP and therefore becomes directly liable for the GP's fee. The fees paid by the CPS have traditionally been agreed with the BMA on behalf of the profession. However, since 1994, the CPS has frozen these payments, and, as a result, these fees are now referred to as 'imposed', to make practitioners aware that they will not be able to seek a higher level of remuneration than that offered by the CPS for assisting in such proceedings.

When called by the defence in a criminal case, a witness enters into a contract with the instructing solicitor. The solicitor will generally seek to offer fees similar to those of the CPS, primarily because the costs allowed will be limited to those authorised by the Lord Chancellor's Department (LCD), through the Legal Aid Board. As in the case of the CPS, the LCD has also refused to increase these fees. BMA members can seek information on the fees paid by the CPS or LCD by contacting their **local** BMA office.

Civil cases

In civil cases where legal aid is not involved, GPs are generally able to set their own fees for undertaking medico-legal work. The actual amount to charge for any professional service can be difficult to decide and should be a matter for individual judgement. The BMA currently (1995) suggests that GPs undertaking medico-legal work may wish to charge between £50 and £97.50 per hour *pro rata* for their professional services. These fees should not be seen as recommended but rather as a general guide that individual practitioners may wish to use in pricing their time. GPs are strongly encouraged to base their charges on a notional hourly rate, rather than simply agreeing to charge 'x' pounds for a particular report, in order to protect their income. In agreeing to write a report, the GP may not be immediately or fully aware of the patient's medical history. It is not uncommon for GPs to spend two or three hours writing what they thought would be a 'brief' report. If they have already committed themselves to a set fee with a solicitor, it is highly unlikely to compensate for circumstances such as these. Agreeing to set their fee in relation to an hourly rate will provide GPs with the necessary flexibility to cope with long reports by retaining the option to charge for the *actual* time it took to complete. As solicitors, accountants and other professionals tend to charge according to actual time, GPs should consider adopting this practice to suit their own circumstances. The BMA recognises that in an era when GPs are facing unprecedented demands upon their time from non-NHS sources and commitments, individual doctors must retain the ultimate discretion of what to charge for calls upon their clinical expertise. Whatever level the GP ultimately decides on, it is essential to communicate this to the instructing solicitor as soon as possible, so that he is aware of likely charges. More importantly, the GP must, in advance of undertaking any work, obtain his *written* agreement to meet these fees.

The only exception to the above is when doctors are appearing in the county courts. Because of the County Court Rules, the sums that may be claimed by GPs appearing in the county court may be severely restricted; for example, GPs preparing medical reports are currently restricted to a fee of between £29 and £57. The fees are so low that they may actually discourage GPs from assisting patients in county court proceedings, and, for this reason, the BMA is pursuing the issue with the LCD to seek a more realistic level of reimbursement for doctors involved in county court actions. It is worth noting, however, that some GPs who have agreed their full professional fees in advance with solicitors have been able to undertake county court work for fees considerably in excess of the county court restrictions. This again signifies the importance of seeking prior agreement for fees with the instructing solicitor.

Coroner's courts

The fees paid to GPs either attending a coroner's court or providing the coroner with a full clinical report are regulated by the Coroner's Act 1988. The fees are generally uprated each year, but responsibility for determining the fees is split between the Home Office, for court appearances, and the Local Government Management Board, for clinical reports. The fees tend to be broadly similar to those paid by agencies such as the CPS. GPs do not have any discretion over whether or not to undertake this work, as they can be compelled by coroners both to attend court and to provide a report. Similarly, while the fees are technically agreed with the BMA, GPs cannot insist on higher payments than those offered for this work.

Payment of fees

It is surprising how many doctors still fail to broach this issue with solicitors until after they have either produced a lengthy medical report or appeared in court. In order to avoid difficulties, it is essential that there is agreement on not only the level of fees, but also a mechanism for paying them. For example, it is hardly worth agreeing to a fee of £100 for a medical report if one is going to wait two years for the account to be settled. The following guidelines should help.

Criminal cases

Payments to doctors should be reasonably straightforward in criminal cases if the GP is instructed by the CPS, as the court itself is generally responsible for meeting these fees, and it is not uncommon for these to be settled within days of a court case. If the GP is instructed by the defendant's solicitors, he may be required to wait until the court case is completed until the fees are met.

Civil cases

In civil proceedings, doctors are generally able to ensure that their fees are paid during the course of a court case, and they should not have to wait until a case concludes. Solicitors acting under the Legal Aid scheme can apply to the Legal Aid Board for prior authority to pay a doctor's fee for a medical report or attendance at court; unlike the CPS, the Board has the ability to make payments on account, and doctors should insist that their fees are settled within a reasonable period, for example one month. If there is failure to agree on a date for payment, the GP may be required to wait for several months for the account to be settled.

Taxation and assessment of witness fees

Doctors should be aware that courts have the power to 'tax' or 'assess' the bills of professional and expert witnesses. Taxation of medico-legal expenses, which is entirely separate from taxation carried out by the Inland Revenue, can result in a doctor's fee being considerably reduced because the court considers his bill to be unreasonable. However, doctors are entitled to seek a prior agreement with the instructing solicitors to the effect that their bill will not be subject to taxation or assessment by the court. By doing so, a doctor can ensure that the fees he initially agrees with the solicitors are the ones he eventually walks away with. For example, if a GP agrees that his fee for attending court is £200 per day (and the solicitor is prepared to accept that these fees will not be subject to taxation or assessment by the court), yet on concluding the case the court decides to reduce his bill to £100 per day, the solicitor will be personally responsible for the shortfall and will still be obliged to reimburse the GP his whole fee of £200. It is therefore crucial that doctors insist, when agreeing their terms and conditions with solicitors, that their fees will not be subject to taxation by the court. Additionally, GPs should not be prepared to undertake work where the solicitor agrees to pay his or her 'reasonable costs'; some solicitors use this as a ploy to engage a particular doctor who, after submitting a bill, discovers that the solicitor does not consider a bill of £100 to be 'reasonable' for a complex medical report. The doctor should always be specific about the actual fee or its likely level and, if necessary, provide solicitors with an estimate, asking them to agree to that fee on the basis of the estimate.

Points to remember are:

- be specific about fee required before doing the work (for example, give an estimate)
- obtain written confirmation of agreement to pay on the understanding that the fees will *not* be subject to taxation or assessment by the court
- do not settle for 'reasonable costs' only – be specific
- if solicitors do not pay, refer them to the Solicitors Complaints Bureau run by the Law Society or consider county court proceedings.

When things go wrong

Non-payment of fees

Attempting to obtain payment for fees will be made all the more difficult if the GP has failed to secure the instructing solicitor's written agreement prior to undertaking medico-legal work. Many GPs still feel reluctant to discuss the issue of fees with third parties, yet, as individuals, they would not consider asking a plumber to install a new central heating system without first discussing the costs involved. There is a lesson here for GPs. A large number of GPs continue to prepare lengthy reports for solicitors, subsequently, attend court and then begin to wonder what fees to charge. At this stage, they are either likely to discover that the fees offered are paltry or be informed that the solicitor cannot or will not settle the account until after the court case has concluded. GPs should therefore be specific from the outset on what they will charge for their professional services (Figure 14.1).

Figure 14.1:   Draft standard letter to solicitors

Smith & Co Solicitors
Anytown
Anyshire
AB1 2CD

Dear Sir/Madam

Medico-legal fees: terms and conditions

I write further to your recent request to prepare a detailed medical report on behalf of your client, Ms A Jones. I set out below my terms and conditions for medico-legal work.

- Reports and qualifying work and conferences with counsel will be based on an hourly rate of £........

- Attendance at court as a professional/expert witness will be on the basis of £........ per half day or £........ per full day.

- Travelling time will be charged at an hourly rate of £........, in addition to travel and subsistence costs.

- If a court appearance is cancelled or rescheduled at less than (*for example 72*) hours notice, I will levy a cancellation charge of (*for example 50%*) of the attendance fee.

Please note that these fees will not be subject to assessment or taxation by the court and that all accounts are to be settled within (*for example 28 days*).
    I would be grateful if you could confirm your acceptance of these terms in writing.
    Yours faithfully

Dr John Brown

Cancellation of the hearing at short notice

This is becoming an increasing problem for GPs who make arrangements to attend court, only to find when they arrive that the court case has been either cancelled, settled or rescheduled without any prior warning. This situation is often further exacerbated because GPs will, more often than not, employ a locum to cover their practice while they are at court. What can a GP do if he finds himself in this position, i.e. without a fee for attending court and facing the prospect of paying for a locum? As a professional witness, the GP is entitled to expect 'reasonable notice' if a case is cancelled or rescheduled. Receipts should be kept to prove that a locum was employed or that a fee had to be paid for cancelling a locum – these can be sent to the solicitors to claim a cancellation fee. The exact amount may vary according to the particular circumstances of each case; however, many doctors tend to use a cancellation charge of 50% of the original court fee. The GP may be able to agree a higher level of reimbursement in the event of a court case being settled or rescheduled; some GPs claim their full costs regardless of the circumstances, and individuals should seek a level that suits their particular situation. The question of what constitutes 'reasonable notice' can be problematic, as it is clearly difficult to introduce a standard timescale for all doctors. In dealing with solicitors, one should ask them for as much notice as possible if any of the court appearance's substantive arrangements are altered. While not encouraging GPs to be overcautious, building in a notice period of seven days will certainly help to focus the minds of solicitors who may require their presence at court and who should be conscious of a GP's considerable commitments, clinical as well as personal. As always, it is vital to obtain the solicitor's written agreement to a cancellation or contingency clause prior to undertaking instructions.

Being served with a subpoena

Being served with a subpoena can be a daunting experience even for experienced GPs. The subpoena, which applies to civil courts, simply means that the court has insisted that the GP's presence is required at court on a particular date or dates. The use of subpoenas is not encouraged, as doctors are usually trusted to attend court voluntarily. However, where a doctor may be involved in a number of court cases, solicitors may seek to obtain a subpoena to 'reserve' him for a particular appearance. Unfortunately, the threat of a subpoena is all too often used against doctors who are unwilling to accept inappropriate fees offered by solicitors for producing reports or attending to give evidence. For example, GPs who have refused to provide a medical report for £30 have been threatened by solicitors with a subpoena, sometimes attempting to infer that, in any circumstances in which a subpoena is involved, a doctor will not be entitled to claim a fee. This is completely inaccurate. While the subpoena may require your attendance as a professional witness, it does not take away your right to receive a fee. Indeed, section 13 of schedule 17 of the Courts and Legal Services Act 1990 makes it clear that a subpoena would be deemed ineffective unless the solicitors who have requested it have defrayed or promised to defray the witnesses' expenses at the time the subpoena is served. For GPs, this can include the cost of employing a locum as well as any travelling (conduct) expenses. While, a GP would technically not be held in contempt of court for failing to attend if the solicitors had failed to pay his reasonable fees, he would be strongly advised to contact the court to make the position known and, if necessary, attend court to explain the situation to the judge.

If threatened with a subpoena, the GP must make sure he informs the solicitors of both his fees and their obligations under the Act. It is clearly in the interests of both doctors and solicitors to maintain a good working relationship, and, wherever possible, the doctor should deal with solicitors in a professional manner similar to that he would wish them to use towards him.

Obligations of solicitors to pay

While we have spoken above about the obligations of GPs, we should not forget that solicitors too have obligations placed upon them. The Law Society, which is both the professional society and regulatory body of the UK legal profession, has set out certain rules to regulate the conduct of lawyers. In the Society's Guide to the Professional Conduct of Solicitors it states that:

> Unless there is an agreement to the contrary, a solicitor is personally responsible for paying the proper costs of any professional agent or other person whom he instructs on behalf of his client, whether or not he receives payment by his client.

This principle applies to fees for reports and other qualifying work, as well as witness expenses. It can be helpful to quote this passage to solicitors who appear reluctant to pay, and it should also help to give the impression that one is reasonably well versed in the conduct of medico-legal work and is aware, therefore, that solicitors cannot simply refuse to pay any fees.

Dealing with former employers: hospitals

It is not uncommon for GPs to be approached by hospitals, as their former employers, asking for medical reports relating to the treatment they may have given to a patient while practising as a hospital doctor. All NHS hospital doctors providing treatment to patients under the NHS are covered by Crown Indemnity. In situations where patients subsequently allege that the care they received was in some way negligent or inadequate, the action will be brought against either the health authority or NHS Trust, rather than against the individual doctor. These requests from hospitals can be frustrating, given a GP's heavy work-load and that he may have left the hospital a number of years previously. As a former employee of a hospital, a GP has no legal or contractual obligation to provide a detailed medical report relating to an incident that may have occurred in the past. A GP would not be obliged to attend court unless the NHS Trust or health authority was willing to meet his fees as a professional witness; however, most doctors will wish to co-operate with reasonable requests for assistance in these matters. If approached by a Trust (a former employing authority) seeking a *factual* report, the GP may wish to consider a reply along the lines of that shown in Figure 14.2.

Figure 14.2: Reply letter to a NHS Trust

Letter to
Anyhaven NHS Trust
Anyhaven
AA1 2HH

Dear Sirs

I am writing to confirm that I was employed as a (*house officer/SHO/ registrar etc*) at Anyhaven NHS Trust between 1990 and 1993. With regard to Mrs AB Jones, I can confirm that I assisted Mr B Green, FRCOG, on 1 January 1992 in the performance of a total abdominal hysterectomy. I would refer you to the contemporaneous notes made at this time for further information.

Yours faithfully

Dr Jane Smith
General Practitioner

Conclusion

Following the advice, and avoiding the pitfalls, mentioned above should help to ensure that dealings with solicitors and courts are enjoyable and relatively pain-free. As with all non-NHS work, unforeseen difficulties may arise. Members of the BMA can seek assistance from their **local** BMA office in dealing with solicitors. However, if the GP has failed to take sensible precautions in agreeing all the terms and conditions in advance, encountering problems should not be surprising. Perhaps more importantly, one should not expect the BMA to be able to put right what one may have failed to do. There is, perhaps, no substitute for experience, and not surprisingly, doctors who have had immense difficulties with lawyers at one stage tend to be more rigorous in their handling of subsequent dealings with solicitors.

15 Opportunities in medical journalism

Tim Albert

Medical journalism is unlike most of the activities described elsewhere in this book. There is no well-established bureaucracy with a statutory need for tasks that only medically qualified people can carry out. It is a free market *par excellence*, in which doctors, perhaps for the first time, will find themselves cast in the unfamiliar role of lay people and competing against experienced professionals for access to a limited amount of space.

Do not be put off. It is also a world in which formal qualifications count for little, and there are good opportunities for doctors (or dilettantes or dustmen) who write well. What is important is whether or not you are willing to understand the needs of the market – and meet them.

Some people find this difficult. They feel that writing is a 'way of letting off steam' or a voyage of self-discovery. They believe that what they have written is an extension of their personality (or, to be more precise, an indication of the excellence of their personality). A request from an editor to delete the smallest adjective becomes a personal affront rather than advice to be heeded. Adherents of this view must understand that they are writing for themselves, and that publication is an added – although unlikely – bonus, otherwise they will have problems.

On the other hand, if you accept that writing is a craft, you stand to derive enormous satisfaction from learning how to do it well. You will have started up the learning curve needed to become a freelance medical journalist. It is unlikely to bring you untold riches: a good rule of thumb is that, at present rates, you will earn between £1 and £2 for every ten words published. It is unlikely to fill your leisure time with boundless fun: most writers agree that the act of writing is rarely enjoyable. However, once published, you should begin to feel an overwhelming sense of achievement. You will be a real writer. You will achieve a certain amount of fame. You may even find yourself being telephoned by editors with urgent commissions or invited to write regular columns. If that happens, you can start to bargain about the pay you receive; you will also feel wanted.

The way of achieving this is easy to describe but difficult to follow: write an article and get it published. The following ten-point guide should help.

1. Select some plausible markets

Many people write first, then look for an outlet afterwards, a tactic that leads to unused manuscripts and bad feelings. Writing successfully is all about making wise decisions, one of the first of which is, for which publications do you wish to write?

Of course, this is easier said than done. Looking around any newsagent will reveal the range of publications available (Box 15.1). You must eliminate

---

Box 15.1:   Markets for writers on medicine and health

- *National newspapers*: feature articles on health pages

- *Local newspapers*: 'A Doctor writes . . .' columns

- *Leisure magazines*: feature articles and problem pages

- *Business magazines:* feature articles on medical aspects

- *Newsletters:* news stories, feature articles and comments

- *Medical newspapers and magazines:* feature articles on personal experiences, articles on clinical practice and opinion pieces

- *Medical journals*: opinion articles (e.g. the *British Medical Journal*'s Personal View)

---

large sections of this and you can only do this if you know what you wish to achieve from your writing. Are you doing it for money, for fame and fortune, for propaganda purposes, or simply for the personal challenge? For whom do you want to write: 'lay' people or those who share your opinions or outside interests? What kind of writing can you do: factual, opinionated, humorous, pompous, political or scientific? More important, what kind of writing can you *not* do? How much time will you be able to spend on it?

When you have considered these questions, draw up a short list of potential outlets. If you wish to improve your technique, but are not interested in money (for the moment, at least), try a parish magazine or a health authority newsletter. If you wish to tell other doctors of the wondrous experiences you have in the surgery, select a GP newspaper. If you wish to communicate to non-doctors, target the health pages of your favourite national newspaper. If you have a hobby, such as stamp collecting or fell running, a specialist magazine may suit.

You may find that your short-list contains some of the publications that you read. These are a good place to start because, as a typical reader, you will be familiar with their style and vocabulary, know the issues that they cover and share their underlying values.

Take your research a step further. It is not enough to know the title of a target publication. Buy (or borrow) several copies. Look at the issues they cover but, more importantly, look for the sections into which your contributions might fit. Many publications have sections for which they actively solicit articles from readers. Be as specific as possible.

2. Define your brief

Once you have a short-list of places where your articles might be published, you can move to the second stage. This involves matching a market with a message, in a process that I call 'setting the brief'.

Ideas are not usually difficult to find: if the worst comes to the worst, open a dictionary and pick a word or two at random. Now develop this idea so that a good message, or 'angle', emerges, suited for a specific place in a specific publication.

To take an example, your idea might be 'difficult patients and night visits'. The subject may excite you enormously, but these two phrases in themselves will not help you to proceed. You need a verb, which will define the relationship between them. For example, 'I hate difficult patients and night visits', or 'Difficult patients always want night visits', or 'Night visits are not the best way of dealing with difficult patients'.

Add the market. Any of the above three might suit the personal view section of a GP newspaper. An alternative piece for *BMA News Review* might be 'Why the system of paying for night visits should be altered because of difficult patients'. Alternatively, for the health page of the *Guardian*: 'How patients can avoid calling doctors out unnecessarily by asking themselves 10 easy questions'.

Put your brief in writing – the back of an envelope will do. Leave it for a while. When you come back to it, throw it some challenges. So what? Is it new? Is it interesting? Will the readers be interested? More importantly, will the editor think the readers will be interested? Is the argument plausible? Are there any obvious loopholes? Is it a fair point? Why me? (The answer 'Because I thought of it first' will usually do, but, in this case, bear in mind that you are writing as a reporter – in the broadest sense – and not as an expert.) Once you are happy that you have a good brief, you are well on the way to becoming a published writer. Therefore, do not worry if this is time-consuming.

3. Collect the information

You may now need to research your article. A common error is over-researching, partly because the reaction of trained scientists is to go to the librarian with a list of key words. They later emerge with a pile of learned papers. This may be a comfort, but rarely advances the task of writing and, in some cases, is a sophisticated form of writer's block.

Research to the brief, not to the subject. What questions does it raise? Answer these directly, which will save you time, force you to think and allow you to cut out information that, although doubtless interesting, is not relevant to your theme. (If the information is that good, you may have the beginnings of your next article.)

If you have to interview someone, declare your interest so that your interviewees realise that their words may appear in print. Agree at the start whether the interview is 'on the record' (in which case you can use whatever they say) or 'non-attributable' (you may use what they say, but not link their name to it). Beware 'off-the-record' interviews: information from these should not be used.

What do you want from each interview – background information or a well-expressed opinion you can use as a 'quote'? You may wish to write down your main questions, but use these as a checklist at the end of an interview, not as a script to follow throughout. Start with some easy questions, such as checking your informant's name and exact title. Ask general questions, and do not be afraid to appear simple and uneducated: the true test is not how you interview but what you write. At the end of each interview, ask if they have anything to add – and make sure that you have a contact number.

Resist the delusion that you will be putting down 'The Truth'. You are collecting evidence to support your brief. Nevertheless, make sure that the facts you cite are accurate. Nothing will ruin a budding freelance career as fast as a misquoted fact, a misspelt name or – perish the thought – a libel suit.

4. Plan an appropriate structure

Articles in scientific journals have their own structure, in which the introduction is followed by methods, then research and finally discussion (IMRAD). It is a curious format, which leaves the interesting part until the end and presupposes a certain amount of commitment among readers (or in reality cares little for them). Writing for other markets demands other tactics.

The way you open will be crucial. Forget about giving the background, or laying out the ground you wish to cover. If you wish to attract passing trade – which is the function of good journalism – your opening few lines must act as a hook for the reader's interest. One of my favourite introductions was written by medical journalist Jeremy Laurance. 'This is a story of sex, fear and money,' he wrote (*Independent*, 29 January, 1991). The article went on to deal with a controversy over the heat-shrinking of prostates, but the way he opened ensured that more people read it than would otherwise have done.

The ending, although important, need not detain you long. If you have written for yourself a good brief, your last paragraph will write itself.

The problem, of course, lies in pulling the reader from introduction to conclusion. In any good writing, a few sentences take the argument forward, while other sentences illustrate or support each point. You can work out which is which by taking a yellow marker pen and underlining the key sentences. If there are too few yellow marks, your structure is weak, and the reader's interest will probably flag. If there are too many, you are trying to say too much too quickly; add a key sentence to bring these points together.

5. Write creatively

By the end of the planning stage, you should have a brief outline of what you want to write. Find some peace and quiet and quite simply start writing. If possible write in one go – this will improve your chances of having a logical flow. When you have written one sentence, move on to the next. Do not contaminate the creative with the critical. Resist the temptation (which some people find extremely strong) to go back and 'correct' what you have written. Resist also the temptation of putting in every detail: at this stage you can add the facts later.

6. Use an appropriate style

Style is a difficult area. It is not a mark of 'personality' or an excuse to show off an expensive education. In the context of medical journalism, it is the choice of words and constructions that best communicates with the target audience. Satisfaction should come from the knowledge of a job well done, of complex matters and arguments understood and explained, and not from decorative flourishes.

Choose appropriate words

Many inexperienced writers feel that, when they sit down at their word processors, they must put on a pompous style. This is not so: the rule is to ask whether you are using the language and constructions you would if talking to your reader in a pub?

Certain principles follow. Do not use a long word if a short one will do: 'start' and 'stop' rather than 'commence' and 'terminate' (Box 15.2). Do not

---

Box 15.2: Pompous words

Avoid	Prefer	Avoid	Prefer
additional	more	apparent	clear
approximately	about	demonstrate	show
elevated	higher	fatality	death
females	women	magnitude	size
participate	take part	performed	did
possesses	has	request	ask
remuneration	pay	reveal	show
stated	said	utilization	use
whether	if		

---

use strings of words, when one will do (Boxes 15.3 and 15.4). Try to avoid clichés, which are tired and unimaginative (Box 15.5).

Box 15.3: Pompous phrases

Avoid	Prefer
as a consequence of	so
at this moment in time	now
considerable proportion	many
due to the fact that	because
general public	people
in addition	also

in the absence of	no
in close proximity to	near
male paediatric patient	boy
members of the medical profession	doctors
reached a conclusion	concluded
substantial number	many
termination of life	death

Box 15.4: Redundancies

(absolute) perfection	(absolutely) unique
during (the course of)	few (in number)
(interpersonal) relationships	(in the process of) visiting
(major) breakthrough	(new) beginning
(skin) rashes	smile (on his face)
(true) facts	worst (ever)

Box 15.5: Clichés

conspicuous by its absence	gold standard
frame of reference	heartfelt thanks
mission statement	more research is indicated
ownership of the health targets	pillar of the establishment
seamless care	state of the art
will be sorely missed	

For a vigorous style, write with nouns and verbs, rather than adjectives and adverbs. 'My next patient was middle-aged, scruffy and objectionable' means little. This is more interesting: 'He was 54, wearing a grey flannel suit that I had last seen in the Oxfam shop just off the High Street. Down the left lapel, next to a thread that meandered down from a button-hole, sprawled the remains of last Thursday's egg'.

Short and logical sentences

Experienced writers sometimes write long sentences effectively. Others generally fail. Keep to about five sentences every hundred words (which is not the same as saying that each should be 20 words). Avoid starting with qualifying phrases ('Following a short discussion caused by the emergency, the decision was made' is better as: 'We talked about the emergency – then made a decision'.) Avoid stuffing one sentence with another as in 'The GP, who earlier in the day had seen 27 difficult patients with conditions varying from tonsillitis to ingrowing toenails and who lived all over the county, got out of bed'.

Use the active voice whenever possible. This means identifying the real subject of the sentence. 'The examination was carried out' is better as: 'The doctor (or medical student or practice nurse) carried out the examination'. 'The debate over night visits is set to be continued by us and particular areas will need to be revisited' is better as: 'We will continue to debate night visits and will revisit particular areas.'

7. Test your writing

Testing your work on others can be a painful process, but it can save countless rejections.

Many people first show their work to their spouses. This is a humbling experience, but will reveal the most stupid of errors. A second person to test your piece on is someone who knows something about the subject (although preferably not the world's greatest expert). A third, and the most important, is someone who represents the readers.

Beware false feedback. Showing a potential *Guardian* article to your colleagues is likely to make it less suitable. Similarly, showing an article for *GP* or *Pulse* to a *Guardian* reader is likely to have the same effect. Apart from choosing your critics carefully, the best way to manage this part of the process is to make sure that you ask each person a specific question, such as 'Will the readers understand?' or 'Have I got my facts right'. Failure to do so will invite a flurry of near-useless minor criticisms.

Throughout this process, remember that you are the writer, and you must take all the decisions. Do not write by committee.

8. Present your writing well

An article is a product like any other, so package it effectively. First impressions are important.

Make sure that you have obeyed – in their entirety – any instructions to authors. If the publication asks for articles on disk, make sure that you comply. If you send 'hard copy' (i.e. written on paper), make sure that it is double spaced, in a good-size type, neatly framed by white space.

Accepting an article from an unknown author requires an act of faith on the part of an editor. Try to make this easier, by attaching a good accompanying letter. This should deal with (1) who you are, (2) what the article is about, and (3) why the editor may find it in his or her interest to publish it. The latter point should be put tactfully; it should not come across as an instruction, such as, 'It's about time you published a decent article'.

9. Present yourself well

As GPs have heartsink patients, editors have heartsink writers, with similar traits. They ask frequent questions, fail to listen to the answers and keep returning for more. Even though your article may have been accepted, you can still ruin a budding career as a writer (Box 15.6). Don't complain

---

Box 15.6: Dealing with editors

DO: Target the right journal
Write in the appropriate style
Ensure that the presentation is good
Keep a copy
Read any instructions to authors
Keep to the required length

DON'T: Argue unnecessarily
Be petty about money
Miss deadlines
Make any mistakes
Send to more than one editor at a time
Send more than one article at a time

---

unless you have good reason. Don't stereotype: ask yourself (or your spouse) why the editor has made a particular change, for instance, and then ask yourself if, in his or her position, you would have made the same. You may be surprised how often the answer is yes.

Throughout, you should give the impression that you are a good professional, who understands the publishing process and can provide the required product.

If you are really unhappy with the subediting, you can ask for your name to be removed. But be careful: I once did this for a distinguished – and allegedly liberal – national newspaper and was never asked to write for them again.

10. Become professional

There are training courses (outlined at the end of the chapter), but there is no substitute for the school of hard knocks and humiliation. Follow up your first piece of work by suggesting a second article for this publication. Your aim should be to build up a relationship with commissioning editors so that they will start coming to you with ideas. At the same time, look for a second market – and repeat the same process. As you do this, you will build your skills and start to develop a network of commissioning editors.

This should not be the end of the story, but the beginning.

Further reading

Albert T (1992) *Medical journalism: the writer's guide*. Radcliffe Medical Press, Oxford.
Evans H (1972) *Newsman's English*. Heinemann, Oxford.
Gowers Sir E (1986) *The complete plain words*, 3rd edn. HMSO, London.
Goodman NW and Edwards MB (1991) *Medical writing: a prescription for clarity*. Cambridge University Press, Cambridge.
Hicks W (1993) *English for journalists*. Routledge, London.
Hennessy B (1993) *Writing feature articles*, 2nd edn. Focal,
Klauser H (1987) *Writing on both sides of the brain*. Harper, San Francisco.
Strunk W and White EB (1979) *The elements of style*, 3rd edn. Macmillan, New York.

Ideas for further training

There are a number of courses on offer to people interested in freelance journalism. This is a personal selection.

Short courses

PMA Associates (The Old Anchor, Church Street, Hemingford Grey, Cambs PE18 9DF, Tel: 01480 300653) runs a wide range of short courses for professional journalism, including a three-month introductory course.

Tim Albert & Associates (Castlebank House, Oak Road, Leatherhead, Surrey KT22 9AU) specialises in short courses in effective writing for health professionals. A one-day course, run in conjunction with BMA News Review, deals specifically with medical journalism.

Longer courses

Many universities and colleges now run full-time postgraduate courses in journalism and shorter courses on specific topics, such as feature writing. The best known are at City University, London; University of Central Lancashire; Centre for Journalism Studies, Cardiff; and Scottish Centre for Journalism, Glasgow.

Correspondence courses:

A number of organisations provide correspondence courses. For an idea of the range, the Monday edition of the *Guardian* is a good place to start.

16   Opportunities in medical education

Eddie Josse

The opportunities available to principals to become involved in medical education have been increasing over the years, not only in the postgraduate field, but also with medical students and other health carers and in non-medical university departments.

The commitment by involved and interested GPs has been considerable, eroding into professional service and domestic time. The financial return has been variable and rarely, if ever, matches the actual work-load incurred. Clearly, it has required the active goodwill of partners and spouses. Female GPs are playing an increasingly important part in the whole field of education.

Many of the opportunities and positions have been recognised by the DoH and have been negotiated through, by or with the support of the General Medical Services Committee (GMSC) of the BMA, leading, in many situations, to the inclusion of explanatory paragraphs in the Statement of Fees and Allowances (SFA) (*see* below). However, many posts, such as academic appointments to undergraduate departments of general practice at medical schools, would not directly concern or involve the DoH.

A perceived advantage of encouraging principals to pursue a high profile in medical education is the positive spin-off that it will have in enhancing primary health care delivery, although it could be argued that it is more likely to be those GPs already providing good quality care who would be prepared and able to add medical education to their professional activities.

The degree to which GPs (and other doctors) have actually trained academically, i.e. for diplomas or degrees in medical or general education, has been variable and generally low, although there is now an almost universal expectation and requirement that teaching courses are attended and re-attended by those involved or wishing to be involved in general practice vocational training.

There is, however, a growing interest amongst GPs in studying for higher examinations, especially masterships in the fields of general practice, community work and education.

Trainers

The activity most recognised by GPs in the field of medical education is that of being a trainer in an approved training practice. This was developed and brought into operation at the same time as the introduction of the NHS in 1948. It came about as a result of an initiative in early 1948 by the then Ministry of Health to, and in the dying days of, the Insurance Acts Committee, the forerunner of the GMSC, some four years before the founding of the college of General Practitioners (RCGP).

Any principal may apply to become a trainer, generally being appointed by a regional general practice sub-committee in England or parallel bodies in the other parts of the UK. Scotland limits the number of trainers who may be appointed at any one time. Each region (or subregion) develops its own criteria and precise administrative arrangements in relation to trainer appointments and re-appointments, although regard is paid to guidelines and a number of expected standards from such bodies as the Joint Committee on Postgraduate Training for General Practice (JCPTGP). Visits to the practice always occur and recur, and regions are constantly nudging up standards. It is expected that GPs on LMCs and local RCGP faculties should be involved in the process of determining standards and appointing and re-appointing their peers.

The commitment by a trainer extends beyond the supervision, teaching and assessment of the trainee. The trainer is expected to attend basic and advanced trainers' courses, trainers' workshops and conferences, take a part in the appointment and re-appointment of fellow trainers, play a role, when requested, in half-day release schemes, and ensure that he or she keeps abreast of training and service developments.

Doctors who are not appointed or re-appointed may appeal against this decision (although not in Scotland) to the GP Trainee Scheme Appeal Committee at the JCPTGP offices (SFA ref: Paragraph 38.1–38.43).

Course organisers

A natural extension of the trainer system was to appoint a trainer with special responsibility to supervise and organise a course local to a number of trainees (registrars), whether in the general practice or hospital phase of training. Thus, the course organiser was born, appointed, as now, through the regional GP advisory machinery accountable to the Regional Adviser in

General Practice (RAGP). Up until 31 March 1992, the remuneration of a course organiser was equivalent to the trainer's grant and was paid via the contracting FHSA out of the general medical services pool set aside for all GP remuneration. Since April 1992, the pay and rations of course organisers became the responsibility of RAGPs acting on behalf of postgraduate medical deans. The global spending on course organiser remuneration, including such costs as superannuation and national insurance, has therefore became part of the postgraduate dean's educational budget, having been deducted in a once-for-all action from the general medical services pool. At the same time, the level of remuneration was greatly enhanced by additional funding (1995/96 = £7922.72, based on two sessions per week), thus exceeding the trainer's grant (1995/96 = £4740.00). The position of course organiser per se does not exist in Scotland; parallel duties are undertaken by Associate Advisers.

It had been recognised that the responsibilities now covered by course organisers had mushroomed to include not only the local scheme educational half-day or full-day courses, but also, for example, setting up and administering three-year vocational training schemes, attending to the needs of trainees on self-constructed schemes, counselling duties, assessment procedures and attending appointment committees, relevant courses and conferences. Most course organisers join their national body, the Association of Course Organisers, which has provided a powerful forum in which to facilitate their development and training. There is no means of appeal against not being appointed or re-appointed a course organiser.

GP tutors

A more recent and welcome development has been the appointment of a cadre of GPs with responsibilities in the area of continuing medical education/continuing professional development in a locality. The appointments were properly recognised by, and funded through, the DoH from April 1993, partly in response to the 1990 contract, although a number of appointments had been made much earlier. The tutors are appointed on a regional (or subregional) basis and are accountable to the RAGPs.

The role of a GP tutor is essentially to try to create an environment in which local principals (and assistants) are encouraged to pursue continuing education and further development. This requires initiative, drive, some understanding of educational processes, innovative ideas, organisational talent and an ability to relate to colleagues and facilitate their own progress.

A National Association of GP Tutors has been formed, and attention has been given to the training needs of new and established tutors.

The remuneration is the same as that for course organisers, and, as for them, there is no appeal against a failure to be appointed or re-appointed.

Regional/associate advisers

RAGPs were originally appointed to develop vocational training for general practice in their regions of responsibility. The GMSC had supported their creation in a policy document of 1968, and an impetus was given to their appointments following the Todd Royal Commission Report on Medical Education of 1968. By the early 1970s, all regions had appointed RAGPs although the original job description of 1972 has expanded to include the financial management of the Section 63 and PGEA accreditation allocations. At this time, continuing medical education for principals was funded through the Section 63 arrangements (of the 1968 Health Services & Public Health Act), administered by postgraduate medical deans, to whom the RAGPs were and are accountable.

It was quickly recognised that, with the expansion of vocational training for general practice in the NHS and its becoming mandatory through legislation by the late 1970s, RAGPs required assistance. By 1973, trainer appointments and re-appointments were being administered through regional educational committees serviced by RAGPs. Throughout the 70s and thereafter, Associate Advisers were appointed, accountable to the RAGP.

The work of an Associate Adviser was and is either on a geographical patch basis or task-specific, for example being responsible for a region's course organisers, GP tutors or assessment procedures for trainees or combinations of these.

Most Advisers hold university appointments, although a few are employed by RHAs. With the disappearance of RHAs and their replacement by the NHSE, new contractual arrangements will be put in place by 1996 to take account of the expanded role of RAGPs in holding budgets for vocational training and continuing medical education. RAGPs have been administering these budgets provided through the DoH for some years. It is, therefore, likely that RAGPs will hold part-time contracts as civil servants for a proportion of their advisory work. They will be looked upon as purchasers of medical education, although many will also have a provider function, largely through the organisation of specific educational programmes.

Regional, Deputy and Associate Advisers are all paid the same remuneration from the commencement of their appointments, namely at the top of the NHS Consultant rate without a merit award. It is counted as officer service and is, of course, superannuable. PAYE deductions are made unless the Adviser is on an NT (no tax) coding, in which case tax is paid in accordance with the Adviser's self-employed status as a GP in contract with an FHSA (or Health Board) and there is a liability for national insurance contributions.

The original intention was that all RAGPs should be part time (working a variable number of sessions per week) and otherwise be principals. A number have become full-time employees and have left active practice, certainly in their capacity as principals. It is clear that the work of RAGPs has expanded very considerably and will continue to do so, with the possibility that most will become full time in the not too distant future. Their additional work includes advising on applications under the prolonged study leave and doctors' retainer scheme arrangements, assisting the GMC in the retraining of doctors with disciplinary or health problems, career counselling, assessing hospital posts for vocational training for general practice, advising the postgraduate dean and other bodies on educational matters concerning general practice, having a role in the development of re-accreditation and developing a relationship with academic departments of general practice at medical schools.

Associate Advisers are part time and likely to remain so. Since they will not be budget holders, there will be no need for them to become civil servants, even on a part-time basis.

RAGPs meet regularly on a national basis, at times accompanied by their Associate Advisers. These meetings and conferences are becoming of growing importance, and, although they are independent of the RCGP, GMSC and JCPTGP, there are links between the advisers and these bodies; for example, RAGPs hold three seats on the JCPTGP.

There is no specific programme of training to become a Regional or Associate Adviser, although most will have had previous educational experience as a trainer, course organiser, GP tutor or member of an undergraduate department of general practice. The main thrust of their work is educational and administrative, although an increasing amount of research is being pursued or commissioned through their departments.

Academic departments of general practice

Although many, if not most, of the appointments to these departments are full time, there are opportunities for principals to be appointed as senior lecturers, lecturers or tutors. The placement of medical students into practices is growing as part of the recognised pattern of enhancing the teaching of medical students in and about the community.

This has in part been recognised as an NHS responsibility, whereby payments may now be made for student attachments in a practice (SFA 40.1 – 40.5).

Other activities

Opportunities exist in other educational fields, such as lecturing not only to doctors, but also to other health care professionals and administrators, for example practice nurses and administrative staff, to members of the public in the St John Ambulance Brigade or British Red Cross Society, and on academic and other courses, for example an MSc or continuing medical education. A number of principals have become very entrepreunerial in arranging intensive courses often linked with leisure activities abroad. It is arguable whether or not the financial return has assumed a higher profile than the desire to provide good educational programmes. However, reports from doctors attending such courses have, in the main, been very favourable.

The PGEA arrangements recognize the educational value of a practitioner's lecturing at an approved educational event by enhancing the credits that can be given to a doctor (SFA ref: Paragraph 37.9).

Conclusion

There is little doubt that there are considerable opportunities enabling principals to become involved in one or more aspects of education (Table 16.1). Remuneration is available, but if doctors look to education as an easy option with rewarding pickings, they would be well advised to look elsewhere.

Table 16.1: Educational opportunities

Post/ experience	SFA reference	Employing/ appointing authority	Usual accountability
Trainer	Para 38	Regional GPS/C or equivalent	RAGP
Course organiser		RHA via GPS/C	RAGP
GP tutor		RHA via GPS/C	RAGP
Regional/associate adviser		University/RHA	PGD RAGP
Senior lecturer, lecturer, tutor Medical student teacher	Para 40.1 – 40.5	University	Head of department
Lecturer, PGEA, other	Para 37.9.	Variable	N/A

GPS/C = General Practice Sub-committee
RAGP = Regional Adviser in General Practice
PGD = Postgraduate (medical) dean

Index